'Till We Meet Again

Melinda Aimée Roth

Dedication

To Mimi (Mignon) Florence Gottlieb Roth

In memory of:

Bernard Roth, Rosalie Chaimovicsova
Rothova, Mor Roth and wife, Berta
Rothova Sichermanova, Martin
Sicherman, and nine children, Serl
Pechterova Rothova

Rifka Gunczenberger Rothova, Lenka Honigova,
two daughters and husband, Helena Rothova, and
Salamun Roth and daughter and wife Leia.

Honoring the survival of Samuel Elias Roth.

May the better gods prevail.

Acknowledgment

Honoring humanity's monitoring of good acts. Wishing for humanity to monitor that evil acts will not happen again.

In tribute to Peter Fabian, Ph. D. who has done the translation of the Czech and Slovakian edition.

Dedication iii

Acknowledgment iv

About the Author vi

About the Author

Melinda Aimée Roth has a Bachelor of Science in biology and has received a later English degree. She has taught in the schools of the Philadelphia School District and has written for newspapers.

Page Blank Intentionally

Partings pained, reunions reigned. Still surviving
made bittersweet existing.

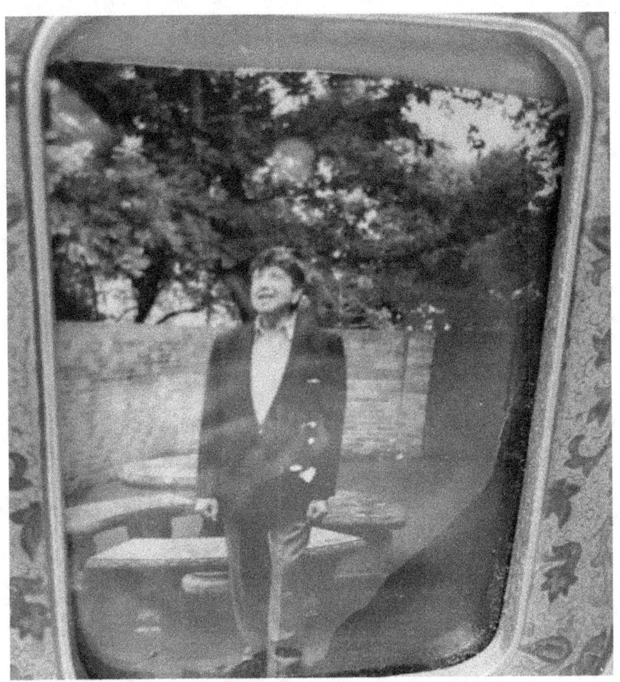

Yet, when the woman was sixteen, her father
had received a letter from his mother, Helen Roth.

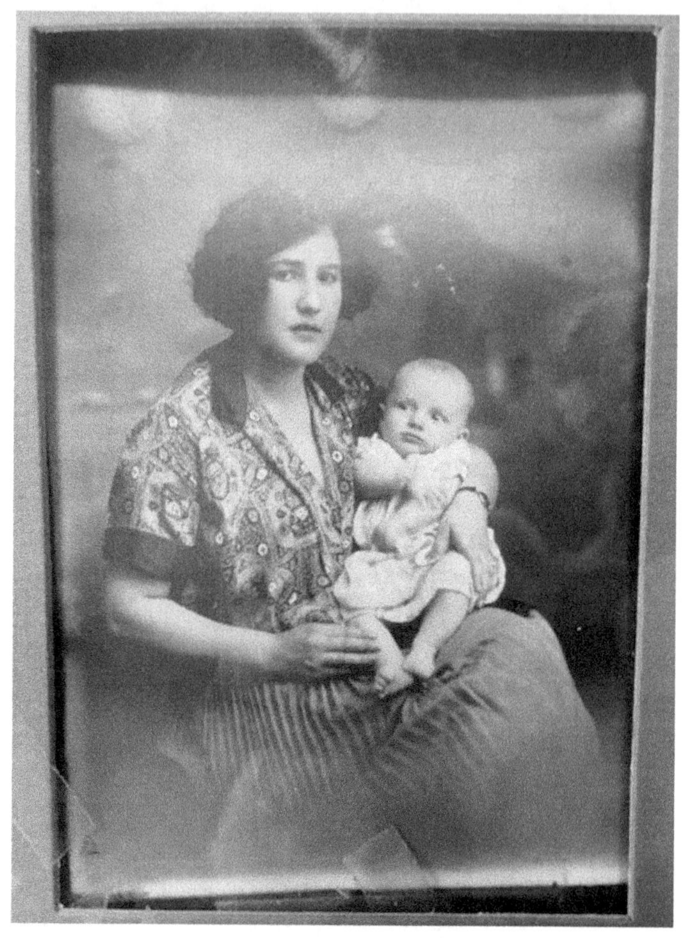

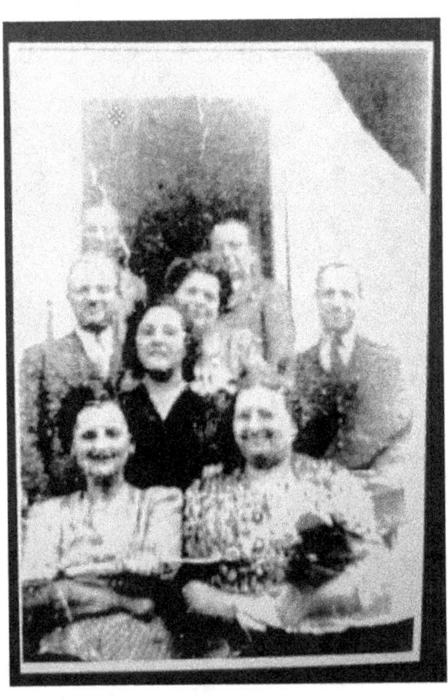

The letter had been sent from Europe to his own mother, Helen Roth, who is in the picture on the previous page and in a black dress above. The picture above includes Yolan Feldman Lang and Regina Lang Roth first row from left to right from the viewer's point of view. Chenshe is in the second row; the third row from left to right is Isadore Roth, Rose Pachter Roth, and Joe Roth, and the top row is Maurice or Morris Lang on the left and Abe Roth on the right top from the viewers' point of view. The letter below was in the language of either Slovak or

Melinda Aimée Roth

Yiddish a dialect of German.

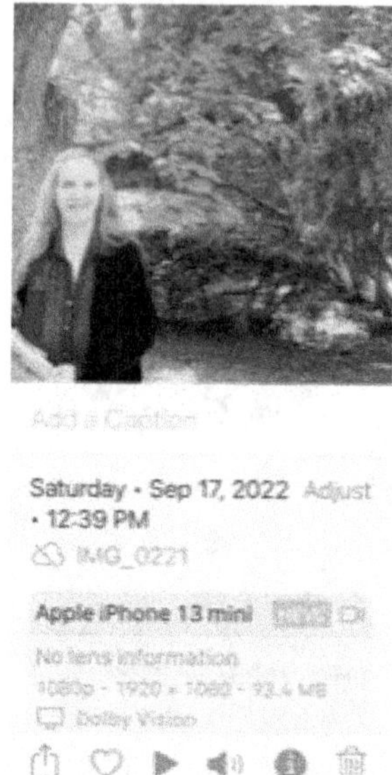

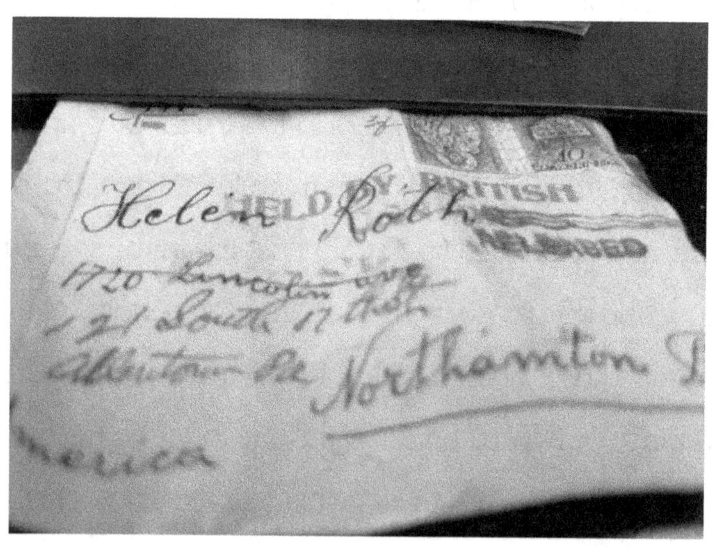

The woman did not have the power, the gumption nor the confidence to walk. . .

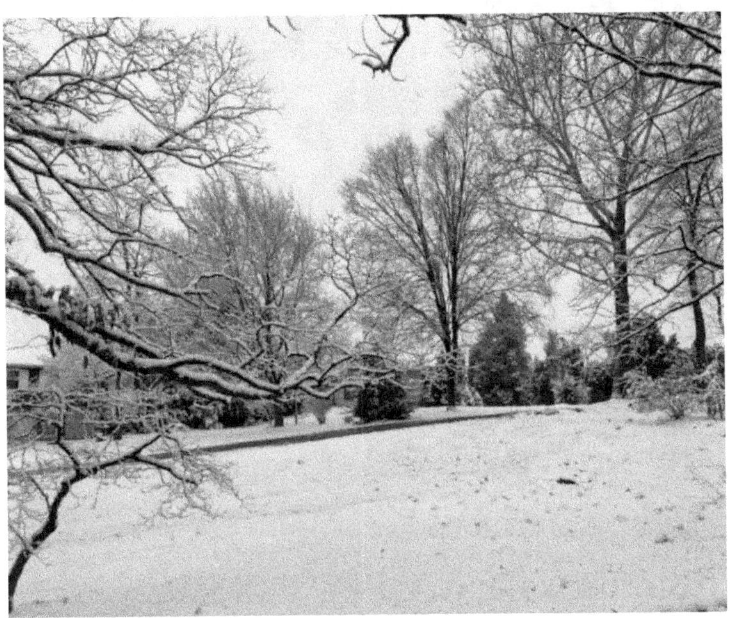

...down the block in Allentown, Pennsylvania, in 1974 as a seventeen-year-old, and thus she could not ask an immigrant family, who lived a block away, for a translation of the letter.

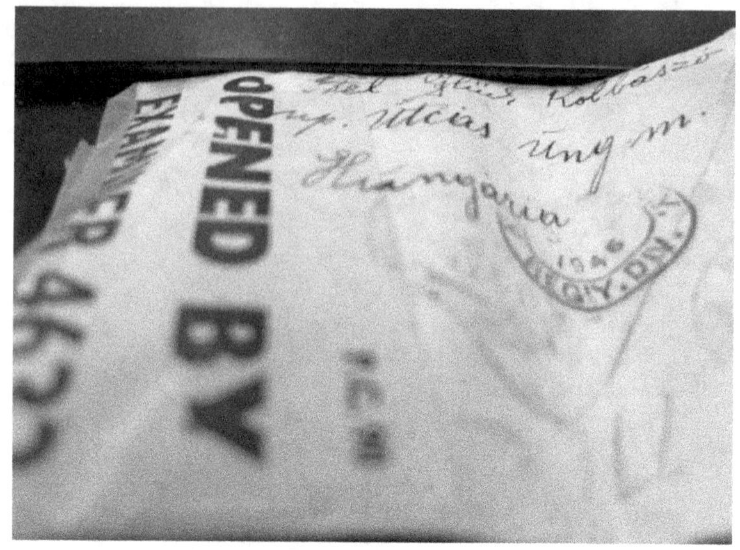

Thus, the letter got lost, but she still had the envelope with the address. Meanwhile, like others, her father was in World War II while his relatives were in dire danger.

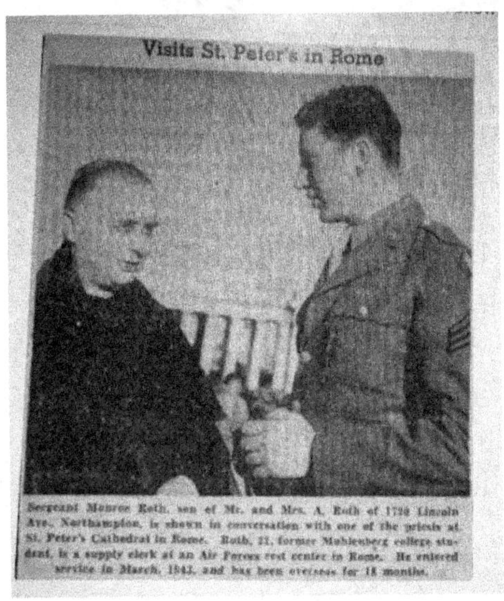

Sergeant Monroe Roth, son of Mr. and Mrs. A. Roth of 1730 Lincoln Ave., Northampton, is shown in conversation with one of the priests at St. Peter's Cathedral in Rome. Roth, 21, former Muhlenberg college student, is a supply clerk at an Air Forces rest center in Rome. He entered service in March, 1943, and has been overseas for 18 months.

Since then, there has been a discovery of an alleged liaison with Yecheil Chaimovics, who is first cousins with the woman's great-grandmother Rosalie Chaimovicsova Rothova.

Yecheil "Charles" Hyman passed away while a resident at his family home on Stanton St. in Hudson, Pa. Mr. Hyman was, for many years, engaged in the meat business. The funeral was held on a Sunday afternoon at 2 p.m.

He arrived in America under the name of Hilly Heimovitz. He was 66 years of age and held for awhile under detention because they thought he was senile. He left behind a son-in-law; H. Majorovic, Nizne Moyne, Czech.

He was headed to philadelphia, Pa. where his son I. Hyman; resided at 325 Spruce St.

He arrived at the port of N.Y. on Oct. 6, 1921, sailing from the port of Antwerp aboard the S.S. Kroonland.

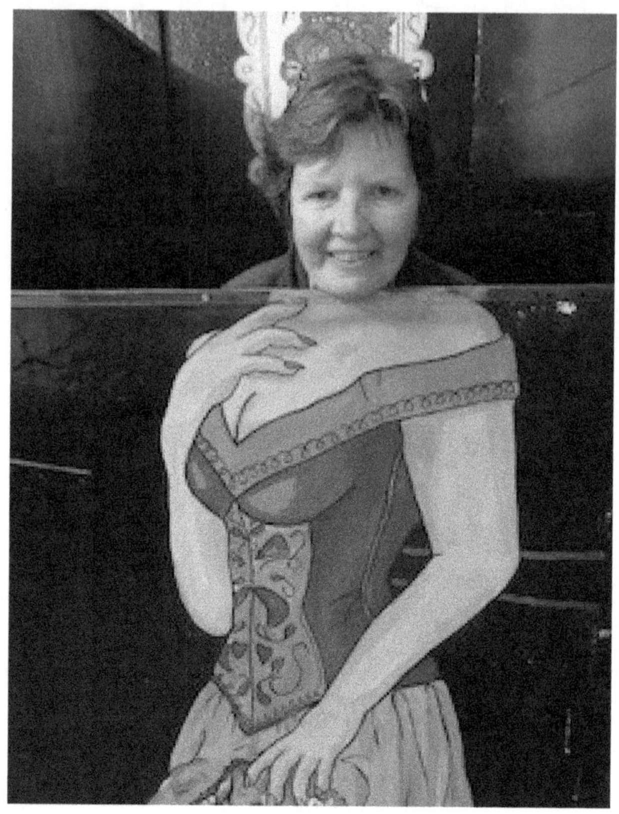

As pictured above, Janet Augusta was studying her relative Sofia who was considered very beautiful.

As Janet managed Zuzana's Ancestry testing, Janet believed that the grandfather of Zuzana was a Roth. But now the theory was either Yecheil Chaimovics or Israel Chaimovics was the grandfather of Zuzana.

These brothers, one or the other, were believed to be the father of Michael Kunco. One of them indeed had had a baby with Sofia in 1896 in Vysna Jablonka.

The name of the baby was Michael. He was
born in 1896.

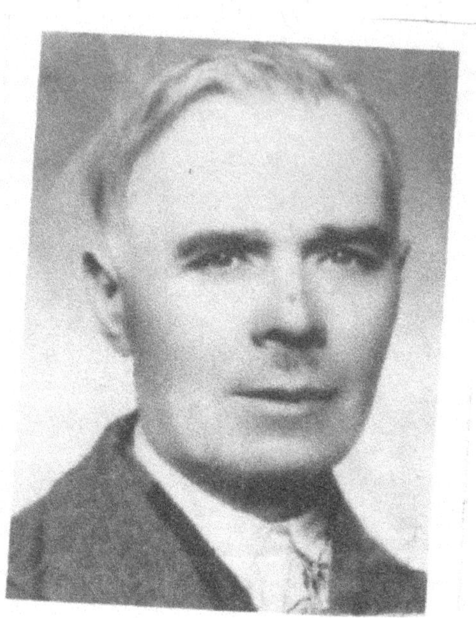

Michael is in the picture above. Michael's
daughter was Zuzana who had tested in Ancestry.
As a result of that test, the woman was contacted as a
match to Zuzana.

Enclosed below is Zuzana in Humenne, at a Slovakian restaurant in 2022. She was 92 years old then.

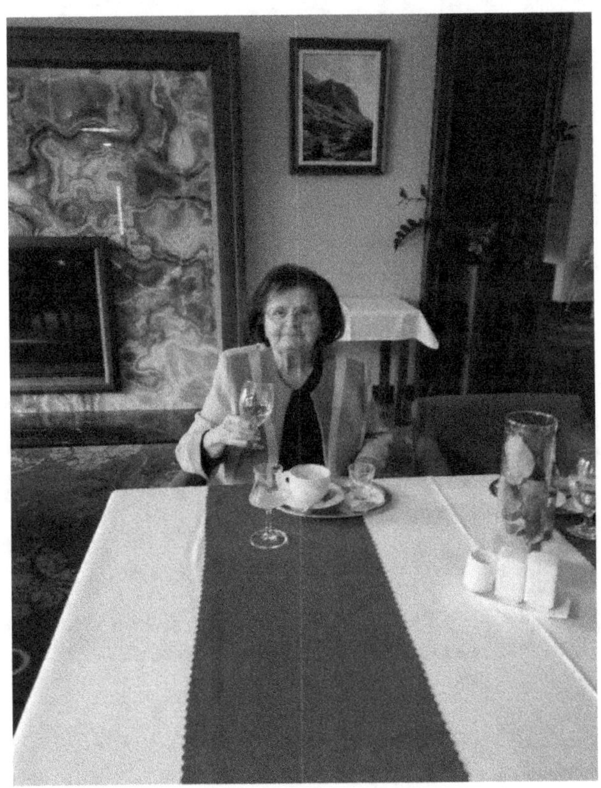

Zuzana has a brother Jan…

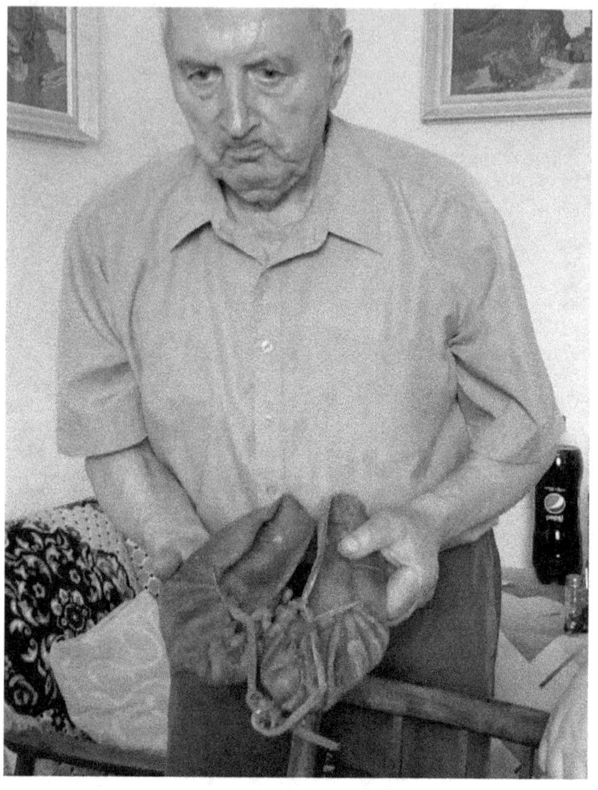

…who lives in Vysna Jablonka as of 2023, and Janet Augusta is a first cousin once removed to Zuzana. Janet Augusta had tested Zuzana with Ancestry.

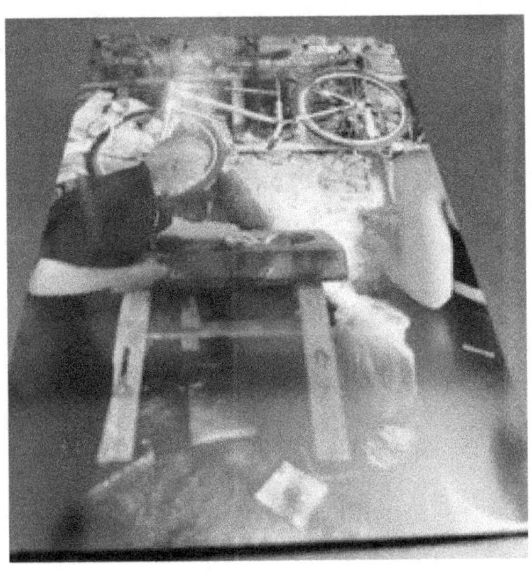

Jan Kunco, in the picture above, in the year 2022, was living in the place of his father, Michael Kunco, in Vysna Jablonka and was showing the milk churn, which was the same milk churn used by his father, Michael Kunco son of a Chaimovics.

Diagram	
Unknown Man	Sofia
Michael Kunco	
Zuzana, Jan	

The woman received the D.N.A. matches of

Zuzana, which is in the largest amounts of identical Centimorgans of D.N.A. to declining amounts of identical Centimorgans between various relatives' D.N.A. and between Zuzana's D.N.A. The highest number of Centimorgans of D.N.A. of Zuzana's as compared to a particular relative's D.N.A. was discovered to be people from the Chaimovics' and the Izcavics' surnames of families on Zuzana's father's side.

The identical D.N.A. between relatives comprises portions of the relatives' D.N.A. that were identical to portions of Zuzana's D.N.A. But recently, there were two people who were highest in identical D.N.A. with Zuzana's D.N.A. They were two granddaughters of Izrael Chaimovics who was the brother of Yecheil.

Diagram	
Izrael	Yecheil
Leah	
Bella, Bozena	

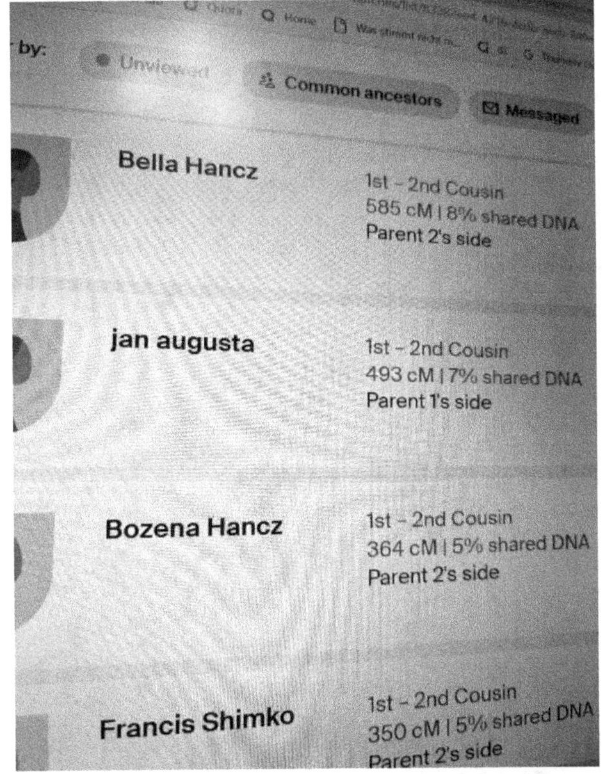

The daughter, Leah, of Izrael Chaimovics, was born to Izrael's wife Rachel in 1897, which was one year after Michael was born from Sofia and from Izrael or maybe from Yecheil.

Diagram
Izrael-Rachel
Leah (b. 1897)

Copy%20of%20Register%20of%20Store%20From%20Vysna%20Jablonka-Rosa%20

bekebelezési engedély és Felső. Jablonka
1799. évi juniushó 11-én kelt adásvevési
szerződés folytán az 1. sztjkönből ide is
jegyzett A †1.002 41. hrsz. si. ingatlanra
a tulajdonjog ténylegs birtoklás alap-
ján.

Kilenczven rénben.
128
1. Chaimovics Hers Leib,
2. Chaimovics Izrael,
Kettő rénben
128.
3. Guzanin Gergely (: kinek neje Czenkó Éva.),
négy rénben
128
4. Csukalovcsák Péter,
négy rénben
128
5. Lukács Mátás (: kinek neje Gula Mária.),
6. Gula Istvám (: kinek neje Ruzinkó Mária.),

To add to this mystery was the discovery of the store register image from the Vysna Jablonka store on the previous page, which had a list in 1899 where the Lukacs family had signed their names. Lukacs was the surname of Zuzana's family, and Izrael Chaimovics also had his name signed on this document in 1899.

One more clue that possibly Izrael was the grandfather of Zuzana is that Izrael lived in Vysna Jablonka and had a deed of property in Vysna Jablonka next to the Lukacs' family's deed of property. Lukacs was the surname of Zuzana's family.

Michael is now believed to be the son of either Izrael or Yecheil Chaimovics and of Sofia. He was born in 1896.

Diagram
Man-Sofia
Michael (b.1896)

With Yecheil, the child would have been born after his wife, Esther Hershovic, had given birth to Yecheil's eight babies.

Again, there was one clue that he might have been a father who had had to leave his child in Slovakia and that was because he had been dazed at the American port in 1921. Another clue was that Yecheil had arrived in America decades later than nearly all of his wife Esther's children had arrived in America.

The question was, was Yecheil love-sick for Sofia, and was this why Yecheil had stayed in Vysna Jablonka much longer than his children had?

Could love sickness go on for twenty years? Indeed, it was now 1921, and Yecheil was having aberrant behavior at a port of entry into America.

Yecheil "Charles" Hyman passed away while a resident at his family home on Stanton St. in Hudson, Pa. Mr. Hyman was, for many years, engaged in the meat business. The funeral was held on a Sunday afternoon at 2 p.m.

He arrived in America under the name of Hilly Heimovitz. He was 66 years of age and held for awhile under detention because they thought he was senile. He left behind a son-in-law; H. Majorovie, Nizne Moyne, Czech.

He was headed to philadelphia, Pa. where his son I. Hyman; resided at 325 Spruce St.

He arrived at the port of N.Y. on Oct. 6, 1921, sailing from the port of Antwerp aboard the S.S. Kroonland.

The write-up above displays how the authorities had retained Yecheil Chaimovics at the American port in 1921 due to Yecheil appearing "dazed."

Within this scenario, to support Yecheil, being the father of Michael Kunco, Esther, Yecheil's wife, would have been forty years old when Sofia allegedly bore Yecheil's child.

Another alternative scenario is that Michael would have been born from Sofia and perhaps another man who did not have a 40-year-old wife, Esther.

Diagram	
Man-Sofia	Yecheil-Esther
Michael?	Annie, Elmore

Still, it appeared that Yecheil's children and grandchildren had also Michael's thin lips, and there were even some redheaded great-grandchildren in all branches of the Chaimovics' family. However, it's important to note that physical appearance or phenotype is not a reliable factor in establishing familial relationships.

Izrael did not have red hair, but he was called "Rot" or "Ishy."

Jana, the daughter of Zuzana, said, "Rot" was for his ruddy skin.

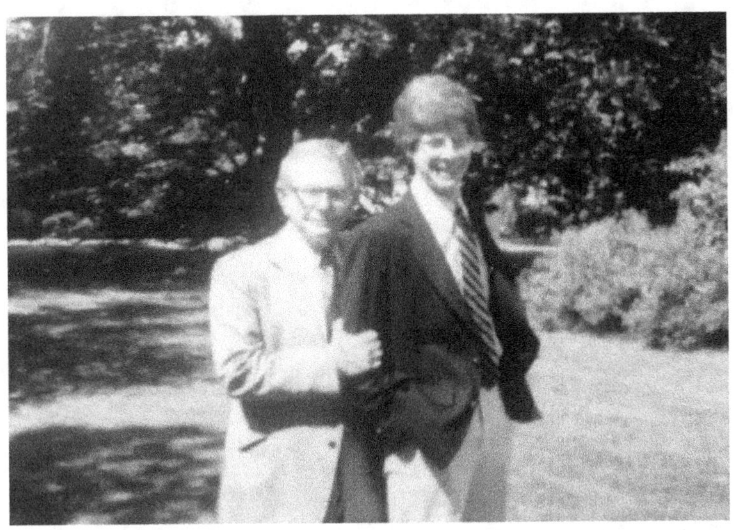

This is Herb, an M. D. and grandson of Yecheil, and Yecheil's great-grandson is Herb's son Nat. Nat has red hair.

Diagram	
Yecheil	Rosalie, first cousins
Elmore-Berta	Abe-Helen
Herb	Monro
R	R,R,R

Herb had one redheaded child, and Monro had three redheaded children.

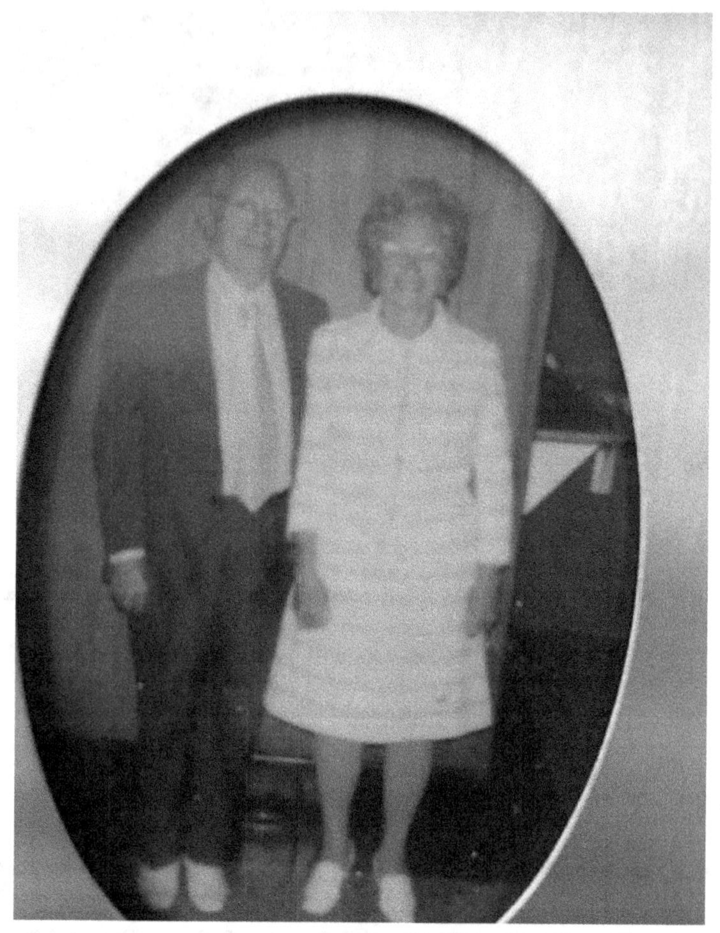

Elmore Chaimovics and his wife, Berta, are in the picture above. Elmore was a grocer, and he did that in Northampton, Pennsylvania, a small town outside of Allentown.

Diagram	
Rosalie	Yecheil
Abe-Helen	Elmore-Berta
Monro,	Herb
3 redheads	1 redhead

Both sides of the two above couples were related, and their grandchildren of both couples had red hair.

Grandpa	
Papa 1	Papa 2
Brother M	Wolf Moskovic
Papa	Samuel Moses Roth
Rabbi M	Helen
Leon, Berta	Lucille

Helen is a third cousin once removed to Berta, the wife, and Abe is a second cousin to Elmore. Both sides of a married couple were related to each side of another married couple.

Diagram	
Yecheil	Rosalie
Elmore	Abe
Diagram-first cousins	
Yecheil, Izrael	Rosalie, Anna
Redheads Are (R)	

Annie	Rosalie	Yecheil
Benjamin (R)	Abe	Elmore
	Monro	Herb
	3 ®	1 (r)

Benjamin Nieman was the son of Annie Chaimovicsova Nieman the sister of Rosalie Chaimovicsova Rothova.

Benjamin became a lawyer who lived in Bethlehem, Pennsylvania. He had red hair. Benjamin Nieman had two sisters, Edith and Berta, who lived later in Allentown. These three were from Annie Chaimovicsova Niemanova who married Mr. Nieman.

Annie, sister of Rosalie Chaimovicsova Rothova, wanted someone to name her descendants after Annie herself, but little did she know that Yecheil, a first cousin to Annie, had a daughter, Annie Chaimovicsova Burnatova, and there were two granddaughters of Annie named Anne.

Diagram			
Annie	Rosalie	Yecheil	
Benjamin	Abe	Annie Chaj. B.	
	Monro	Child, Child	
		Annie, Anne	

Diagram	
Yecheil	Annie
Annie	Benjamin
Child, Child	
Anne, Anne B.K.	

The one granddaughter, Annie Burnat Kellman, was the first clue in Zuzana's D.N.A. matches that Zuzana's Jewish grandfather was a Chaimovics and not a Roth.

So, Annie, Mr. Nieman's wife, gave her name to a first cousin's two great-granddaughters in a way. Also, Annie had a son, Benjamin Nieman, who had red hair.

Annie was the sister of Rosalie Chaimovicsova Rothova and a first cousin to both Yecheil and Izrael.

Benjamin Nieman the son of Annie Chaimovicsova is in the picture below.

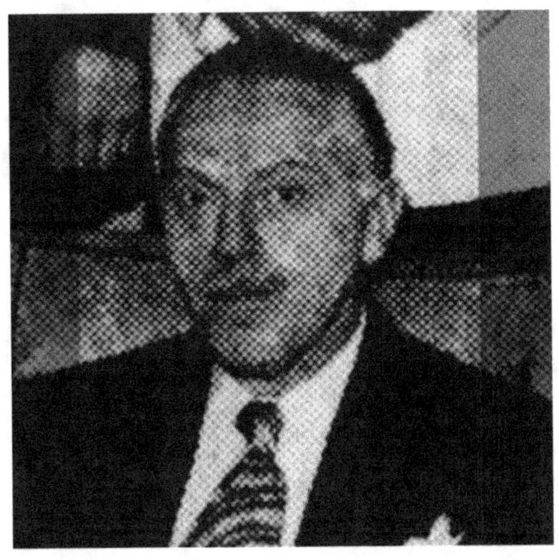

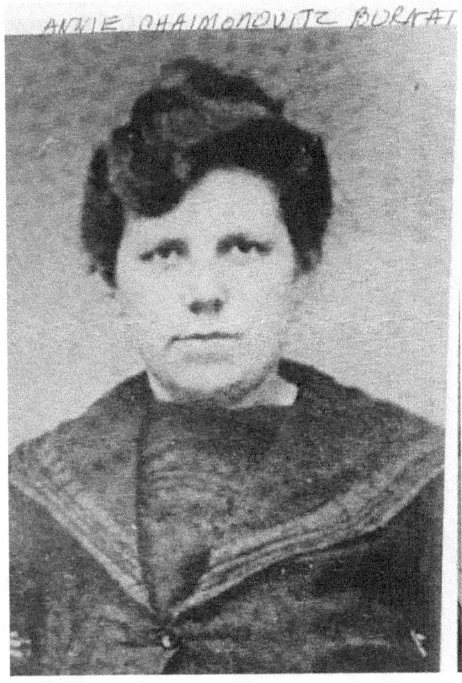

Annie Chaimovicsova Burnatova, pictured on

the above page, was the daughter of Yecheil and had
thin lips, as did Elmore a son of Yecheil.

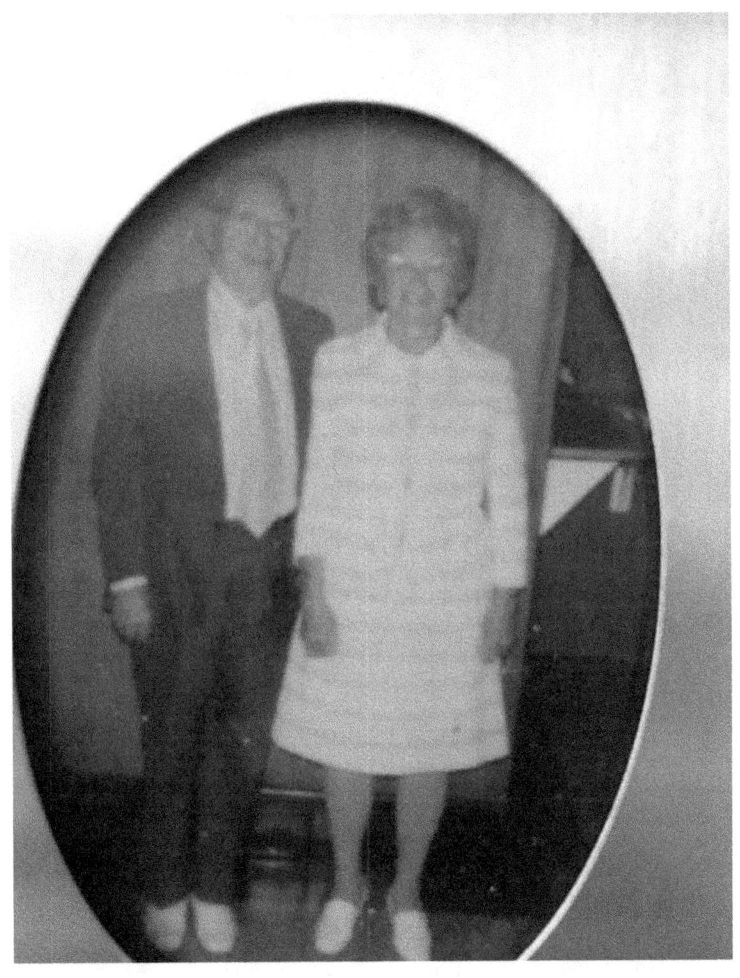

Elmore and Berta are above. Michael Kunco
may have inherited his thin lips from Yecheil, as it
appears to be a physical characteristic shared by both
of Michael and Elmore.

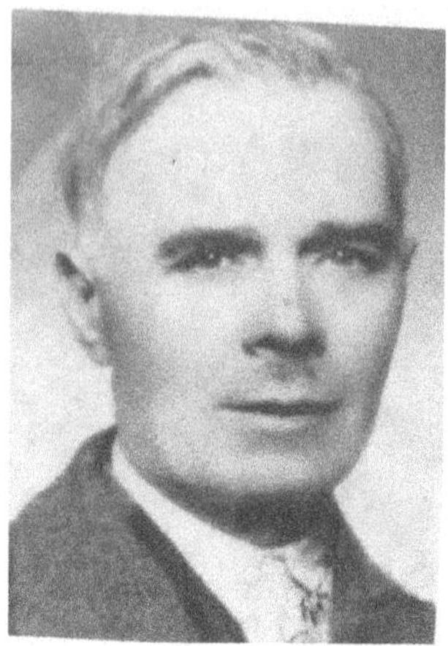

Michael Kunco, who had thin lips, is shown above and was either the son of Izrael or of Yecheil Chaimovics.

Annie Chaimovicsova Burnatova had 14 children and then died at a very young age of 55 years of age. She had lived outside of Scranton, Pennsylvania.

Diagram
Yecheil
Annie
14 Children

Joan Roth Lichtenstein said that Saturday evening was the day for relations, and it was an honor to have one baby per year, but every other day was a day where one worked hard. Also, families began having babies when the mother was approximately thirteen years of age, according to Ann Burnat Kellman's cousin, Ron Tiso.

Diagram	
Joshua	Bernard -Ros.
Jacob	Abe, Joe, Isador
Joan Roth Lich.	Monro

Izrael Chaimovics, Yecheil's brother, had never left Slovakia. The store where he worked was in Vysna Jablonka. But Zuzana said her grandfather, either Yecheil or Izrael had owned a farm and a forest, had worked with horses, and had worked in the store, and finally had left for the United States.

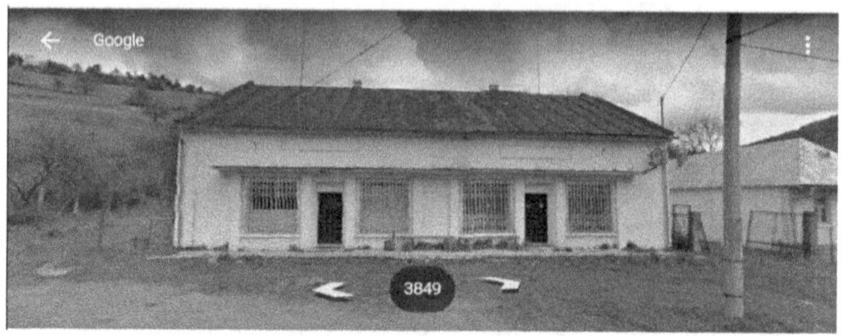

In fact, Zuzana says her grandfather patted his son Michael who was Zuzana's father. The grandfather of Zuzana left for what was said to be the other country; Zuzana said either Yecheil or Izrael immigrated to the United States. The farm where the entire family lived in one room is located below and also has Kata Jr., who served as a translator for Melinda in 2022, pictured in it.

The picture from left to right from the viewer's point of view is:

Jan's cousin, and Jana; Ursula, who is blond; Vlad, Sona, and Kata, Sr. in the front row from left to right from the viewer's point of view. The farm is in Vysna Jablonka in the year of 2022. The farm is the farmhouse of Jan Kunco brother to Zuzana.

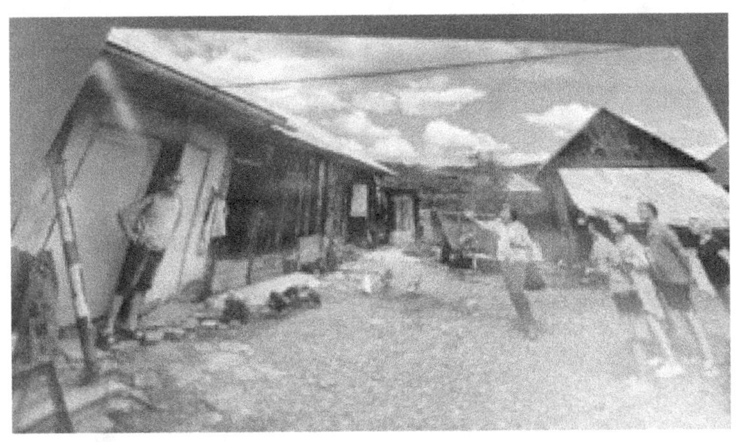

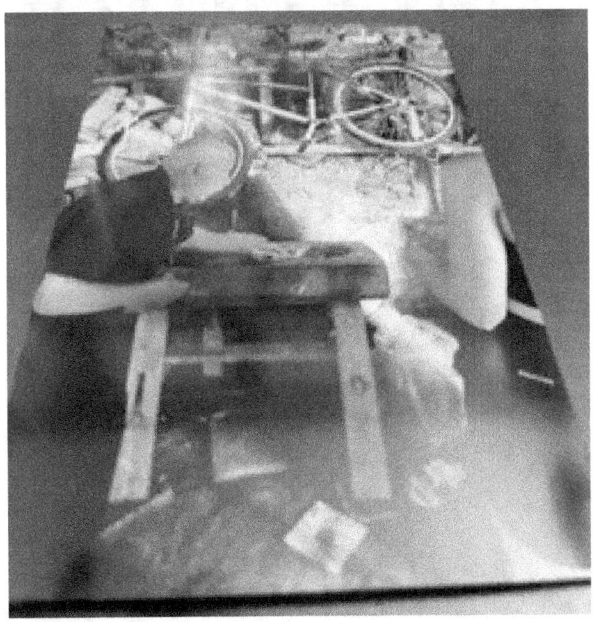

When the D.N.A. was taken of Zuzana, the
highest number of Centimorgans identical with a
relative's portion of D.N.A. had recently been Bella,

Izrael's granddaughter who had 585 Centimorgans identical to Zuzana's D.N.A.

Bella's D.N.A. is 99% marked as Jewish and 1% marked as Greek and Albanian. Certain markers within the D.N.A. can indicate a person's country or ethnic origin.

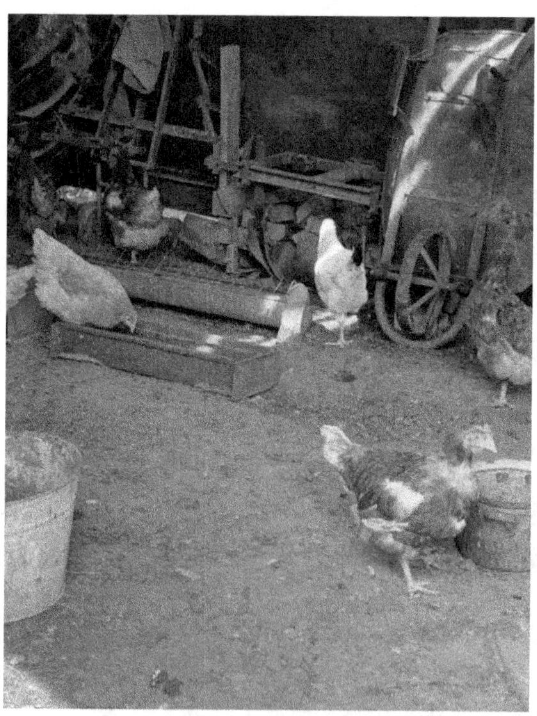

The land on the previous page is where Michael Kunco had lived in Vysna Jablonka, and now his son

Jan lives there in 2023. Jan is the grandson of a Chaimovics due to a clue of Anne Burnat Kellman's D.N.A., a granddaughter of Annie Chaimovicsova Burnatova. Anne Burnat Kellman tested highly as a D.N.A. match with Zuzana's D.N.A.

Diagram	
Man-Sofia-	Yecheil-Esther
Michael	Annie Chai. B.
Zuzana	Man
	Anne B.K.

Ann Burnat Kellman's D.N.A., being a high match to Zuzana who is the granddaughter of Sofia Kunzco or Kunco, was the first clue that Zuzana's grandfather was a Chaimovics.

Additional clues can be found in the relatives who are Roths outside of the Chaimovics-Roth family bond and who did not match Zuzana's D.N.A., such as Judith Roth, born in Cluj, Romania, as well as Vicky Schulkin and Anita Lindenberg

Myers.

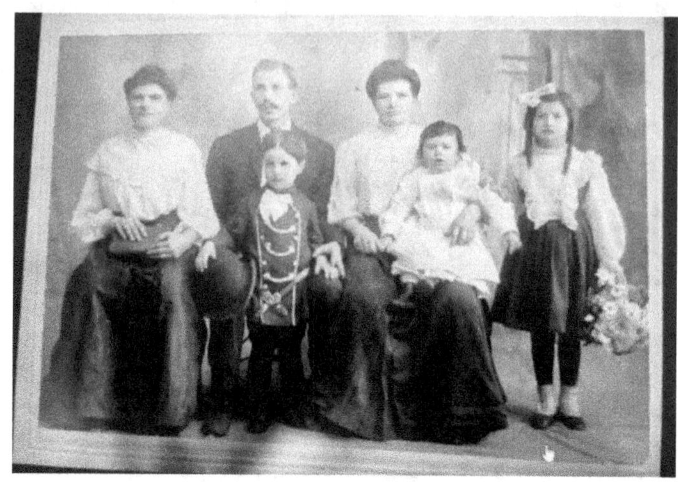

Rose Roth, the woman with the baby on her lap in the picture above, is the grandmother of Anita. Anita is second to third cousin to a grandchild of Abe and Helen Roth; Anita is a Roth outside of the bond with a Chaimovics. The picture was taken in about 1920 in Brooklyn. Rose's granddaughter, Anita, did not match with Zuzana.

The list of D.N.A. for Zuzana's D.N.A., matches relatives' portions of Zuzana's D.N.A. The portions of Zuzana's D.N.A. are identical in that portion to a particular person's portion of D.N.A. are as follows:

1) Bella's D.N.A. is highest as a match to Zuzana's D.N.A., in the amount of 585 Centimorgans.

2) Bozena's D.N.A., which is on the same parent's side as Bella's D.N.A., is Bella's sister's D.N.A.; Bella is another of Izrael's granddaughters with 364 Centimorgans of D.N.A. identical with Zuzana's D.N.A. which Ancestry.com surmises has a 73% chance that Bella and Bozena are half first cousins to Zuzana which is what the case would be if Izrael be Zuzana's grandfather.

Diagram	
Rachel-Izrael-	Izrael-Sofia
Leah	Michael, Mary
Bella, Bozena	Zuzana, Helen
	Jana, Francis

Zuzana and Francis, who both took the test, would be first cousins once removed. A new discovery has been made in Francis, who shares 350 Centimorgans of identical D.N.A. with Zuzana's D.N.A. Ancestry states that there is a 70% probability that Francis is a first cousin once removed from Zuzana, as indicated in the diagram.

Diagram	
Rachel-Izrael-	Izrael-Sofia
Leah	Michael, Mary
Bozena, Bella	Zuz., Helen

Francis is the child of Helen and a first cousin once removed from Zuzana. Francis's D.N.A. composition has the same ethnic composition as Zuzana's, which perhaps explains that Francis, born in 1939, is a descendant of Sofia. In fact, Francis, the grandson of Izrael's daughter Mary, is also from Sofia.

Diagram	
Rachel-Izrael	Sofia
Leah	Michael, Mary
Bozena, Bella,	Zuzana, Helen

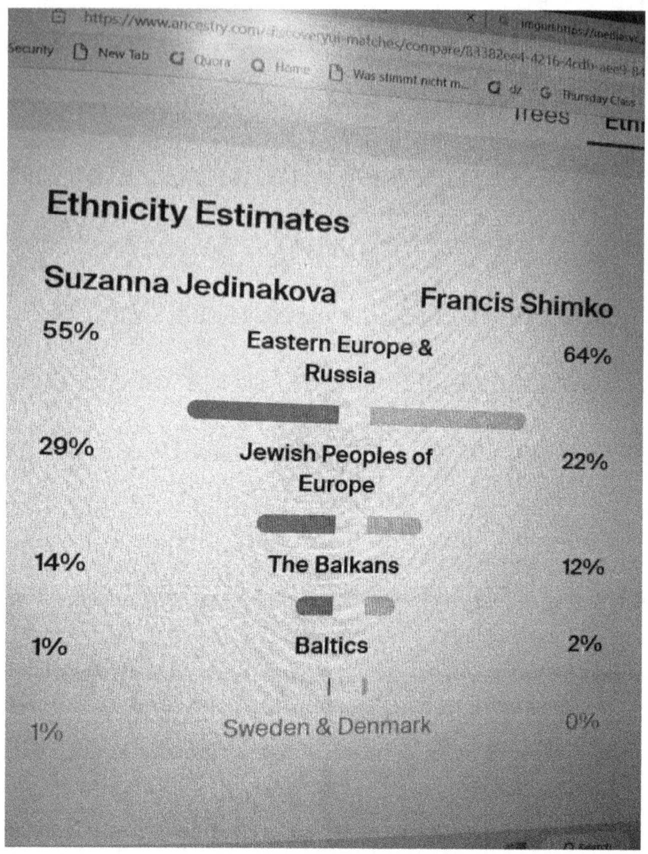

The D.N.A. list of a person also provides the identical D.N.A. Centimorgans between Zuzana's D.N.A. and the person's D.N.A. listed. The list also provides the ethnicity and the percentage of chance of a particular relationship between the two people.

Ancestry.com provided this ethnic composition of Zuzana's D.N.A. due to her D.N.A. being tested and by the D.N.A. of Francis, who also was tested.

Izrael-Sofia	
Michael	Mary
Zuzana	Helen
Jana (Tested.)	Francis (Tested)
Jana-65E.E.	Francis-64E.E.
E.E.=% Eastern European	
Jana 12 J.	Francis 22 J.
J.=% Jewish	
Jana 16 B.	Francis 2 B.
B.=% Balkan	
Jana=7 Balt.	Francis 2 Balt.
Balt. = % Baltic	

The above is the ethnic composition of two people in the same generation, both Ancestry tested.

The variability could be due to the generations

above in the diagram with different partners' D.N.A. and their ethnic composition.

Diagram	
Izrael-Sofia	Izrael-Sofia
Mary-partner	Michael-partner
Helen-partner	Zuzana-partner

Izrael has 100% Jewish- marked D.N.A., and Sofia is 100% Christian- marked D.N.A., or Sofia might have some Centimorgans of Jewish- marked D.N.A.

Michael, their child, has 50% Jewish- marked D.N.A., and Zuzana, the following generation, the daughter of Michael, should be 25% Jewish- marked D.N.A... But Zuzana is 29% Jewish-marked D.N.A. on the Ancestry list of Zuzana's D.N.A., and variabilities could happen partially due to partners' D.N.A. having Centimorgans of that ethnic composition.

Diagram		
Rachel-Izrael	Izrael-Sofia	Izrael-Sofia
Leah	Michael,	Mary
Bella, Boz.	Zuzana	Helen
	Jana	Francis

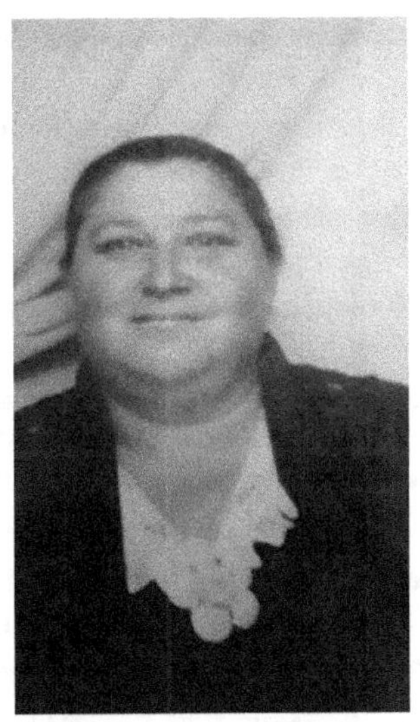

The above is Mary Kunso, the daughter of Izrael
Chaimovics. The spelling of the surname is slightly
different. One could notice Mary's thin lips. Mary
lived in the United States and somehow was brought
from Slovakia and was discovered through the

D.N.A. to be related to Zuzana. Mary's grandson Francis was tested, and the manager of the D.N.A. was interviewed and stated that Mary Kunso was the grandmother of Francis. Mary was found to be the daughter of Sofia and of Izrael through the calculations of Centimorgans of identical D.N.A. with Zuzana who was tested.

Izrael-Sofia
Mary
Helen
Francis

Diagram	
Rachel	Israel-Sofia
Leah	Michael, Mary
Bozena, Bella	Zuzana, Helen
	Jana, Francis
Leah	Mary, Michael
Bella, Bozena	Helen, Zuzana

<table>
<tr><td></td><td>Francis, Jana</td></tr>
</table>

If one goes up one generation in the family tree, the Centimorgans double, resulting in a 700 Centimorgan match between Zuzana and her first cousin, Helen.

The Deoxyribonucleic Acid (D.N.A.) is like a double-stranded necklace with "beads" on it. The "beads" are in pairs.

In each cell in one human, the D.N.A. is located in the nucleus of each cell. Millions of cells are in one person, and all of the cells have a nucleus with the D.N.A. inside each nucleus per cell.

With the same order of "beads," the D.N.A. creates a template for the R.N.A. or Ribonucleic Acid like a single-stranded necklace located in the cytoplasm of each cell of one human. This process of D.N.A. and then R.N.A. is for a process to make proteins.

Again, the order of "beads" in the R.N.A. has the same order in every cell of one human.

If a person infected with the coronavirus is within six feet of an unmasked healthy person, the virus, which contains R.N.A., can enter the healthy person's cells through his or her membranes of cells. Once inside, the virus takes over the healthy person's cellular R.N.A. machinery and can cause the person to become sick.

Based on other scientists' work, this D.N.A. knowledge was also worked out in the 1950s by Scientists James Watson and Frances Crick. The vaccine is a piece of deadened R.N.A. of the Virus that will elicit antibodies to fight the illness.

Yet in the village of Vysna Jablonka lived Zuzana.

As of 2023, Zuzana lives in Humenne, a bigger town near Vysna Jablonka. She is now 93 years old as of the year 2023 and lives with her daughter Jana as of March 2023.

Zuzana always knew that she had a Jewish grandfather. Her brother Jan always knew and was embarrassed at times with differences. There also was a taboo with people of various religions getting married or reproducing together. Zuzana has 29% Jewish -marked D.N.A. So, Michael has 58%, and Izrael can only have 100, so the 8, which is doubled, comes from Sofia.

Genealogist George Pappas, and relative to Janet Augusta, explains this in a way-"Francis has 350 Centimorgans with Zuzana. According to Ancestry.com that is correct-so Helen has 700 with Zuzana. That is conjecture... when a child receives exactly 50% of his D.N.A. from each parent, further generations don't each receive exactly 50% in the same way. Helen and Zuzana are first cousins once removed, which means that they should share anywhere from about 102-980 Centimorgans." He then states that Mary and Michael should have 1613 to 3488 Centimorgans as full siblings. He believes that they are full siblings.

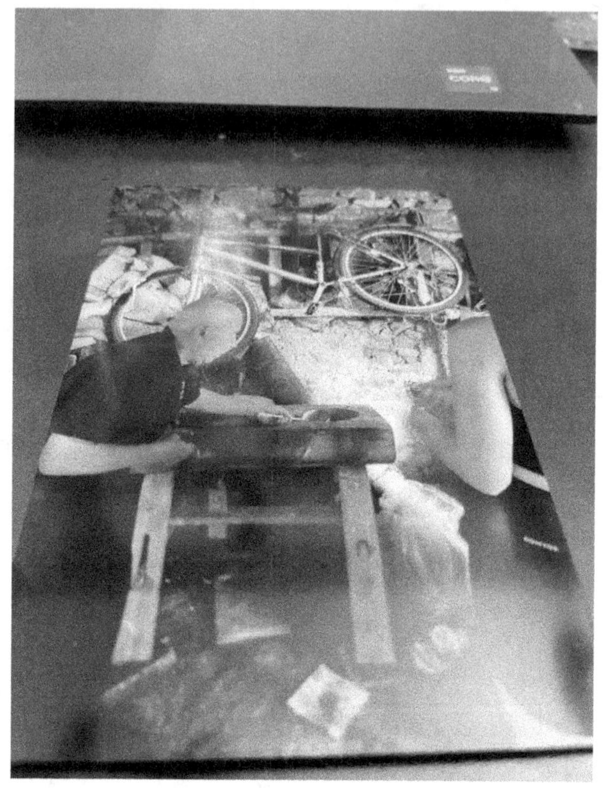

Jan works in a barn and is the brother of

Zuzana, and both have a Jewish grandfather, Izrael

Chaimovics or Yecheil.

In the D.N.A. matches of Zuzana is a highly

matching man with his D.N.A. and he is named

Dan.

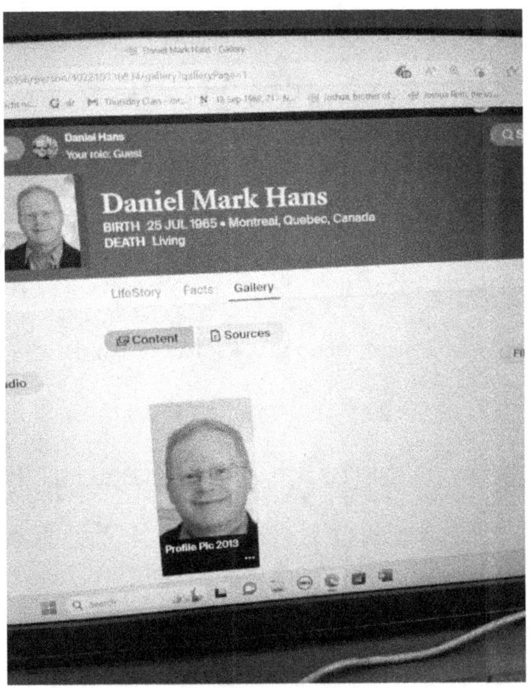

Dan is the nephew of Bella and Bozena. He, when interviewed, explained about two aunts in their 90s. The two aunts were D.N.A. tested. Dan also told of a great-grandfather, Izrael Chaimovics, from Vysna Jablonka. Dan also has red hair. Daniel claims that his great-grandfather Izrael never left Vysna Jablonka. Daniel is a great-grandson of Izrael.

After the recent discovery of the 1930 Czechoslovakian Census, provided by

JewishGen.Org, it is now known that Izrael was living in Humenne in 1930. The Census listed Izrael living with his son Jakub Chaimovics born in 1904 in Vysna Jablonka. Jakub is a son of his wife and is on the Census, as well as Jakub's parents-in-law and brother-in-law and also a widowed relative, Rosalie, born in 1913, who was born in Vysna Jablonka and was living with them. It was discovered that Izrael's wife, Rachel, had passed away in 1925. Due to his presence in Humenne of this list during the 1930 Census, it is clear that Izrael did not immigrate to the United States at that time.

**Searching for Surname (phonetically like) : CHAIMOVIC AND
Any Field (contains) : HUMENNE
7 matching records found.**
Run on Mon, 17 Apr 2023 19:00:32 -0600

Sheet # House # / Family #	Name Birth Surname	Birth Date Birth Town	Relationship	Comments	Box Year Reference
0385 260/2	**SICHERMAN**, Albert	07-Feb-1865 Pavlovce	head		
0385 260/2	**SICHERMAN**, Johanna	Mar-1870 Velke Zbince	wife	married 10-Mar-1891	
0386 260/2	**SICHERMAN**, Ludvik	20-Sep-1905 Trstany	son		
0386 260/2	**CHAIMOVIC**, Jakub	11-Apr-1904 Vysna Jablonka	son-in-law		0258 1930 SNA Bratislava ludu 1930
0386 260/2	**CHAIMOVIC**, Malvina	05-Jan-1901 Trstany	daughter	married 18-Jun-1929	
0386 260/2	**CHAIMOVIC**, Izrael	16-Feb-1858 Vysna Jablonka	co-father-in-law		
0386 260/2	**CHAIMOVIC**, Rosalia	29-Dec-1913 Vysna	relative	widowed 1924	

Izrael had a daughter Leah, who had two daughters, the already mentioned Bella and Bozena, who all had emigrated and had gone to Canada.

Both sisters took the Ancestry test and matched very highly with Zuzana. In fact, Bella matches with 585 Centimorgans of identical D.N.A. and has 99 % Jewish -marked D.N.A. and 1 % Greek and Albanian- D.N.A. with Zuzana.

Sister Bella matches with 364 Centimorgans of D.N. A. identical with Zuzana's D.N.A. So, both sisters have high portions of identical D.N.A. with Zuzana's identical portions of D.N.A.   A cousin once removed to Zuzana is Janet Augusta who has 100 % Christian -marked D.N.A. Janet Augusta is related on Zuzana's maternal side.

Yes, the D.N.A. has markers resulting from evolution and can indicate a) culture, b) country, and c) religion due to tribes, religions, cultures, and countries where people have been reproducing within exclusive groups for thousands of years.

Below is Jana who is a retired judge and the daughter of Zuzana.

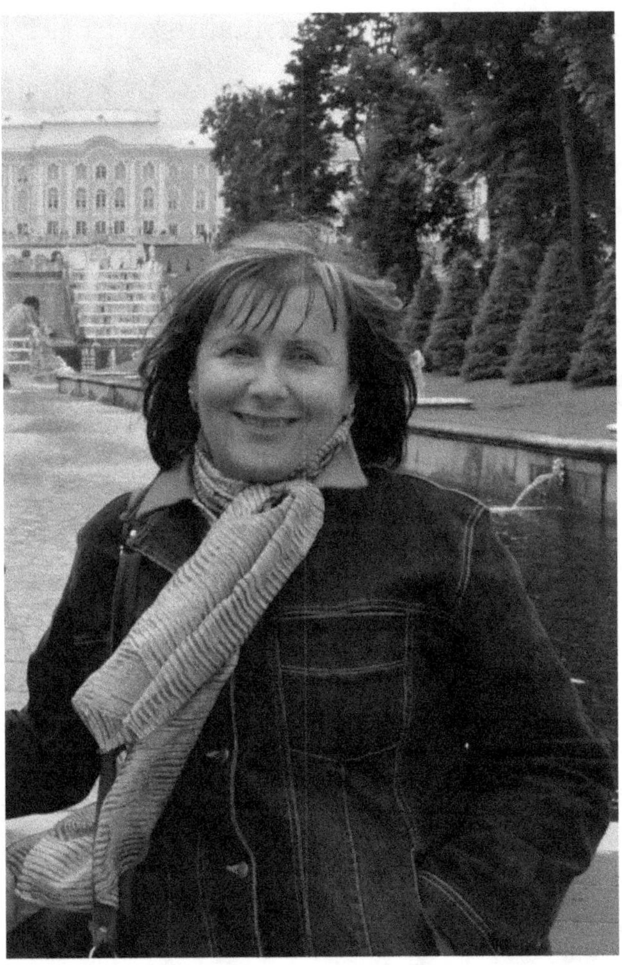

According to oral testimony by Jana, Zuzana's daughter who is a retired judge, there was a man who came to get eggs and sheep and brought the eggs and sheep back to Humenne, a larger town, in 1896 when there were horse-driven carriages. In fact, Jana, the daughter, says there were no cars in Vysna Jablonka until the 1970s.

The barn is where either Izrael or Yecheil Chaimovics used to come to get eggs and bring them back from the tiny village of Vysna Jablonka and take the eggs to Humenne in Slovakia. The man taking care of the barn now is Yecheil's or Izrael's grandson, Jan Kunco.

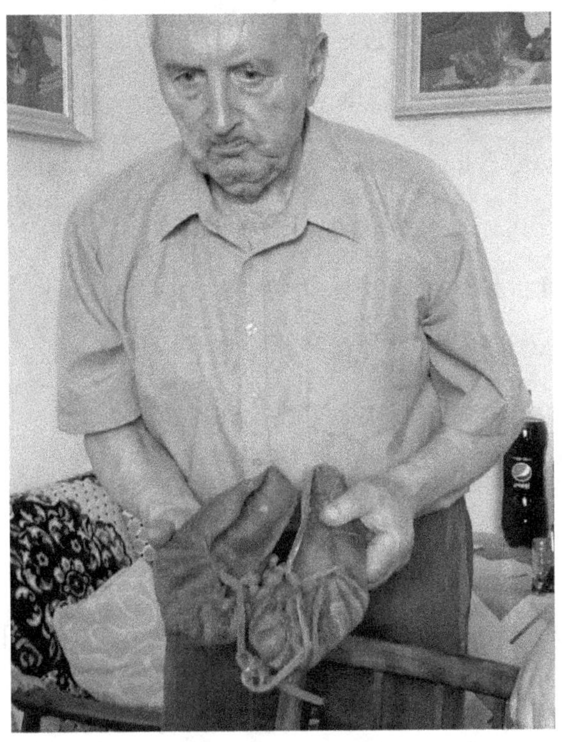

Jana is the daughter of Zuzana. Zuzana's grandmother Sofia was the mother to many children, some of them foster. According to Janet Augusta, Sofia was supposedly beautiful, and her husband had gone to America immediately before the liaison occurred between Sofia and either Yecheil or Izrael Chaimovics. Janet also says that Gregorius Gula, Sofia's husband, had passed before this liaison.

A baby boy named Michael was born in the village in 1896, followed by the birth of a baby girl named Mary in 1900. Mary was the mother of Helen, and Helen was the mother of Francis who happenstance took the test and discovered his past. Mary was in the United States. She apparently was brought over by Sofia Metrik another Sofia who was a relative of Sofia Kunco Gula.

After Sofia Gula may have passed in 1902 at 44 years of age, the baby must have been handed over to Sofia Metrik, whose name was changed to Rose Picker who may have traveled for the military according to Ancestry's documents.

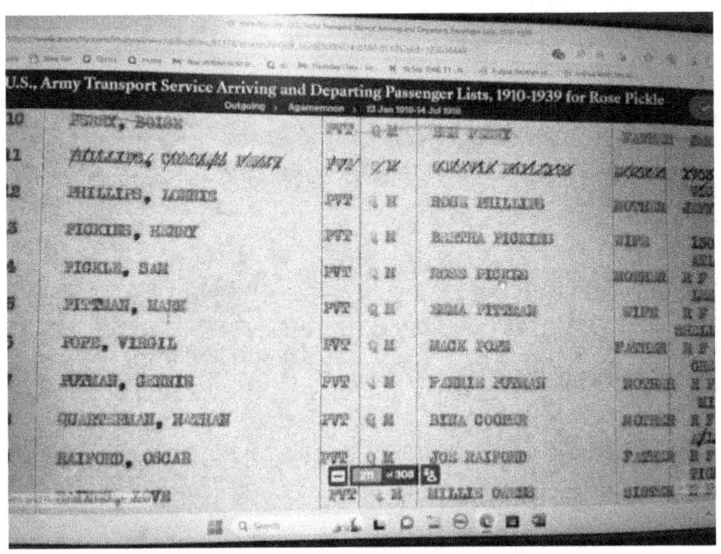

Sofia's parents raised Michael, Jana said, and the village knew that Michael had 50% Jewish marked D.N.A., actually 58%. The 58 %, one figures out because the daughter Zuzana has 29% Jewish-marked D.N.A., so she gets half from Michael. If Michael has 58, he can only get 50 from Izrael's 100 % Jewish -marked D.N.A. Sofia has 16 % Jewish-marked D.N.A., which gets halved with her children.

Michael's and Mary's half-sister was Leah.

There was a son of Izrael, Jakub Chaimovics born in 1904 to his wife Rachel, who is on the 1930

Czechoslovakian Census. Izrael was living with Jakub's family and with a sister-in-law widowed in Humenne, Rosalia Chaimovicsova.

Sofia, Izrael's liaison, passed in 1902, according to documents where there is no longer writing about her. In 1930, on the Census, Izrael did not have his wife, Rachel.

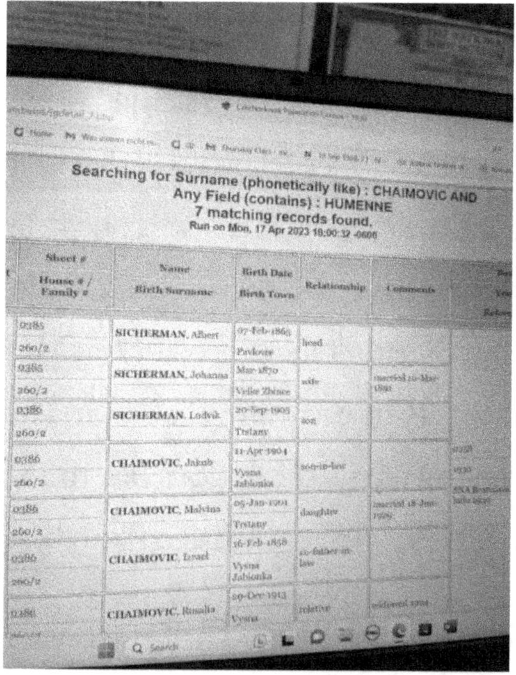

Searching for Surname (phonetically like) : CHAIMOVIC AND
Any Field (contains) : HUMENNE
7 matching records found.
Run on Mon, 17 Apr 2023 18:00:32 -0600

Sheet # House # / Family #	Name Birth Surname	Birth Date Birth Town	Relationship	Comments	
0285 260/2	SICHERMAN, Albert	07-Feb-1865 Pavlovce	head		
0285 260/2	SICHERMAN, Johanna	Mar-1870 Velke Zbince	wife	married 10-Mar-1891	
0386 260/2	SICHERMAN, Lodvik	20-Sep-1905 Trstany	son		
0386 260/2	CHAIMOVIC, Jakub	11-Apr-1904 Vysna Jablonka	son-in-law		
0386 260/2	CHAIMOVIC, Malvina	05-Jan-1901 Trstany	daughter	married 18-Jun-1929	
0386 260/2	CHAIMOVIC, Izrael	16-Feb-1858 Vysna Jablonka	co-father-in-law		
0386 260/2	CHAIMOVIC, Rosalia	10-Dec-1913 Vysna	relative	widowed 1930	

Zuzana daughter of Michael was tested, and all Chaimovics who tested with Ancestry now match with Zuzana's D.N.A. Also, the Izkavics family distantly matches with Zuzana's D.N.A., who are one generation back from the Chaimovics. The Izkavics include Rock Star Leonard Kravitz and Actress Deborah Winger.

Yecheil had a wife Esther Hershovic whose seven children went to Scranton, Pennsylvania, United States, decades before Yecheil finally went to America in 1921.

Hershovic, Weisberger, and Berkovic were originally Schmulkovic. All three brothers, in the mid-1850s, changed their surnames and walked in different directions to avoid conscription, but that is another story.

Meanwhile, in 1896, Yecheil Chaimovics was married to his wife, Esther Hershovic, and by 1921, his wife, Esther Hershovic, was 40 years old and no longer had any children with Yecheil.

Yecheil Chaimovics, who was married to his

wife Esther Hershovic, remained in Slovakia for several decades after seven of his eight children had left for the United States. This raises the question: was Yecheil a love-struck man who couldn't bear to leave his homeland despite his family's departure?

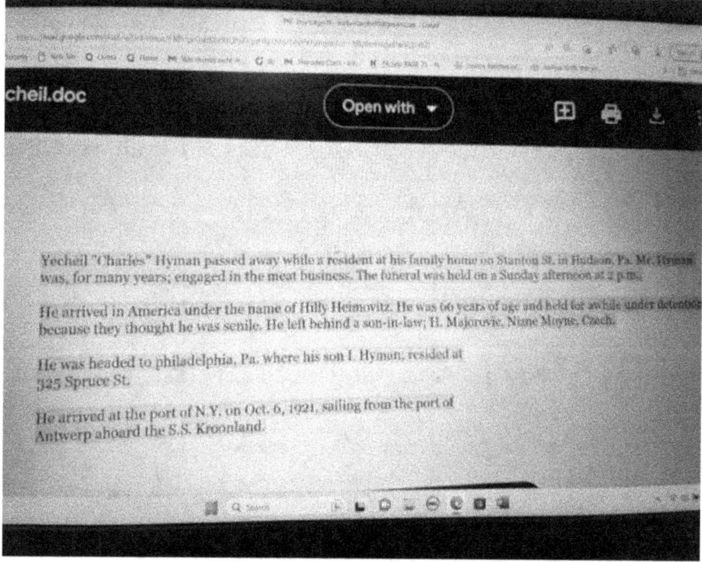

cheil.doc

Open with

Yecheil "Charles" Hyman passed away while a resident at his family home on Stanton St. in Hudson, Pa. Mr. Hyman was, for many years, engaged in the meat business. The funeral was held on a Sunday afternoon at 2 p.m.

He arrived in America under the name of Hilly Heimovitz. He was 66 years of age and held for awhile under detention because they thought he was senile. He left behind a son-in-law; H. Majorovic, Nizne Moyne, Czech.

He was headed to philadelphia, Pa. where his son I. Hyman, resided at 325 Spruce St.

He arrived at the port of N.Y. on Oct. 6, 1921, sailing from the port of Antwerp aboard the S.S. Kroonland.

Yecheil was dazed and confused and held in detention at the port in 1921 in New York.

One child of Yecheil's remained in Humenne named Hermina who had worked in the small store with her descendants. The descendants, Peter and

Sister, are grandchildren of Hermina. The grandchildren left Humenne in the 1970s and are living in Canada as of 2023.

An important fact of this story is that Yecheil or Izrael came to say goodbye to Sofia and patted the son, Michael, on the head, according to Zuzana. The man was the father of a baby with Sofia. Sofia is Zuzana's grandmother.

Yecheil, on the ship's list to America, called himself a "Merchant." At the port in 1921, he was "dazed" and held there in New York City.

Diagram	
Sofia-Yecheil-E	R.-Izrael-Sof.
Michael, Mary	Leah
Zuzana, Helen	Bella, Bozena

The woman wanted to maintain her belief that Yecheil was the grandfather and not Izrael. However, despite the revelation from the granddaughter she states that the grandfather did leave the country. Izrael never did leave Slovakia, and calculations keep indicating that Izrael is the father of Mary and Michael.

With Yecheil as their grandfather, Zuzana is second cousins to Bella and Bozena, which is not what Ancestry says. Izrael is the father, of Leah and of Michael and of Mary. Bella and Bozena are both half-first cousins with Zuzana and Helen, just as Ancestry says.

Diagram	
Rachel-Izrael-Sofia	
Leah,	Michael, Mary
Bozena, Bella	Zuzana, Helen
	Jana, Francis

Yet Izrael never left Slovakia, and the granddaughter Zuzana says her grandfather came to say goodbye to his son Michael, Zuzana's father. Is it possible that Izrael was saying goodbye because he was going to Humenne with his son Jakub?

Bella, Bozena	Zuzana, Helen

Now, there is another development. Rosalie or Roza Chaimovicsova Rothova or Roza Rothova is the older woman in the picture below. The man in the white hat, Joe Roth, traveled to Slovakia from Allentown, Pennsylvania, in 1936, and thus the picture was taken.

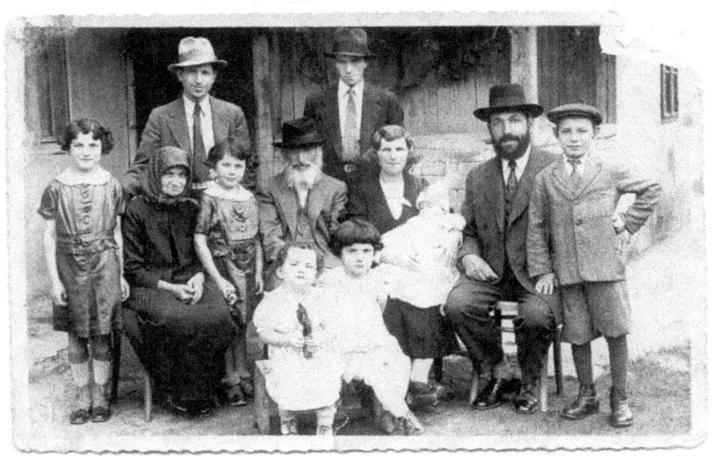

The man in the black fedora in the back row was discovered to have survived Auschwitz; he was discovered by American relatives in 2019 to have been an Auschwitz survivor living in the Czech Republic. His name was Samuel Elias Roth, and he was born in 1912.

Samuel was the son of Jakub Roth son of Bernard Roth. Jakub passed in 1915 before his parents Bernard Roth and Roza Rothova, passed.

Diagram	
Bernard	Roth-Roza Chajmovicova
Abe, Isador, Joe, Jakub, Berta	

Abe, Isador, and Joe went to Allentown, Pennsylvania, by the 1920s.

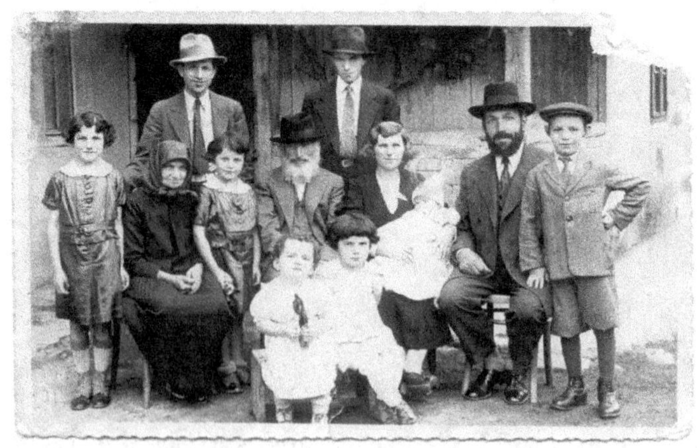

Samuel Elias is in the black fedora next to his uncle Joe Roth with a white fedora in the picture- both are in the back row. Joe tried to convince his parents, Roza Chaimovicsova Rothova and Bernard Roth and Berta, his sister and family, and his nephews Samuel Elias and Moric and wife Katerina, to immigrate to the United States. Still, all remained in Europe after Joe Roth had traveled to Slovakia in 1936.

Joe in the white hat had traveled in 1936 to see his family; he had come from Allentown, Pennsylvania and tried to convince his family to leave. He returned to Allentown, Pennsylvania, and told his daughter Adele Roth Wolensky, "Something bad is happening there." Then Adele told the woman, "They did not expect what would happen."

Samuel Elias Roth, the man in the black hat in the back row, came back to Vysna Jablonka in 1946 after having been in Auschwitz and did not find his relatives, and so he went to Teplice, Czech Republic, with his "army buddy," said Alex's granddaughter.

Samuel Elias Roth then wrote a letter in Slovak or Yiddish a non-mainstream dialect of German, to relatives in Allentown, Pennsylvania. Still, no one knew who Alex Roth, Sr. was. Samuel Elias Roth had changed his name. Monro was the son of Abe, and Abe was the son of Bernard Roth.

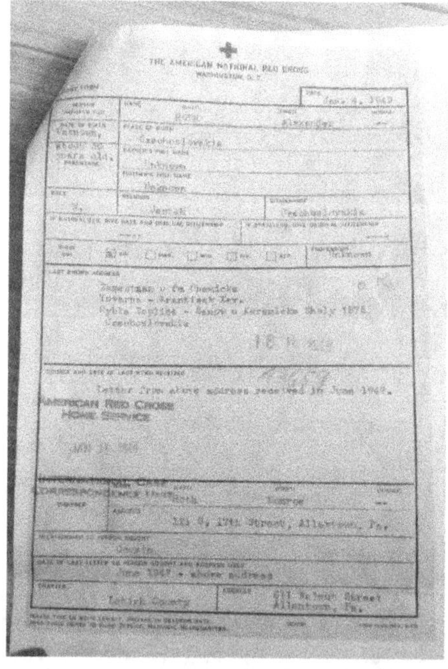

Monro had just finished serving in the Air Force during World War II.

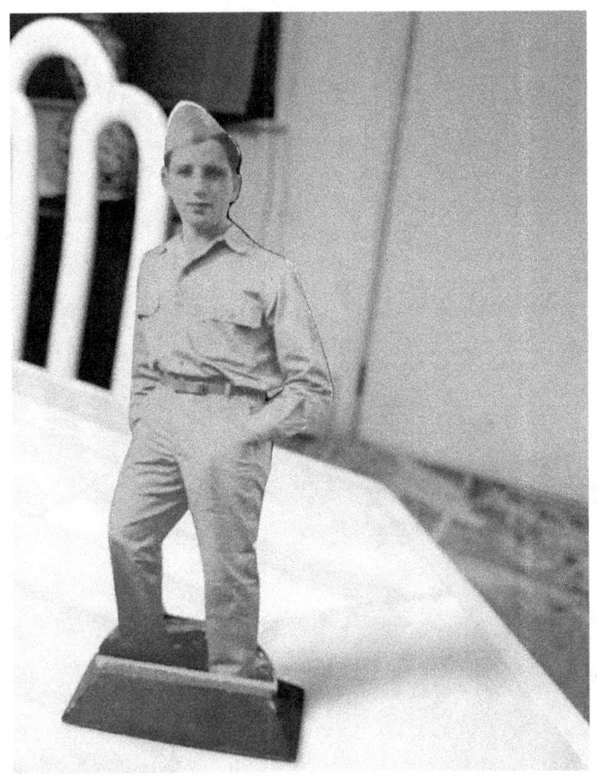

The picture above is Monro Roth. Monro filed a document in 1947 with the Red Cross to find Alex, Sr., or Samuel Elias. Samuel Elias's granddaughter, Sona, found the document in 2019 and wrote a letter to Monro's survivor Lucille Roth Lehrich on Facebook in 2019.

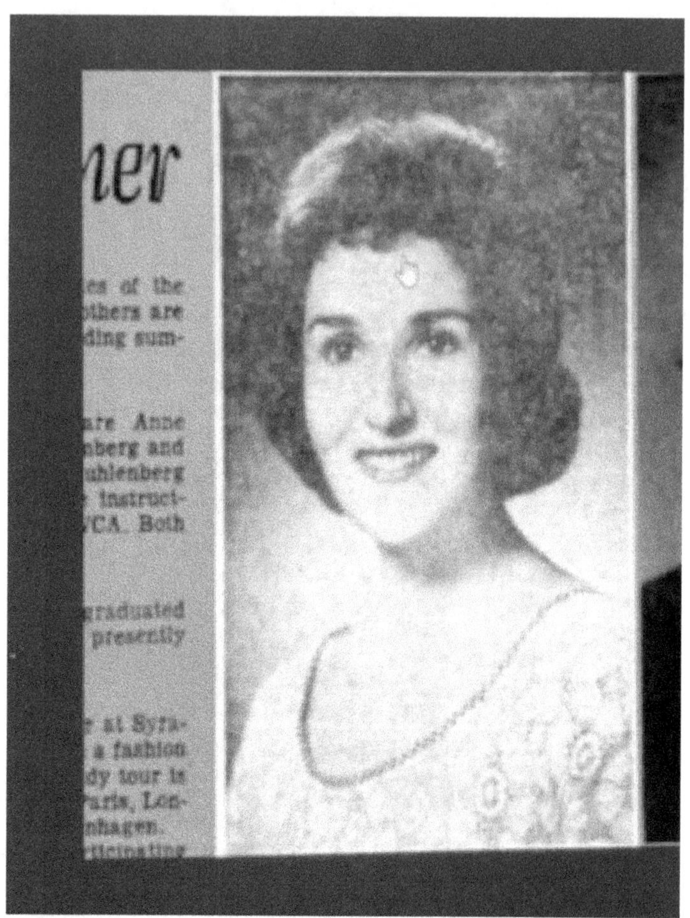

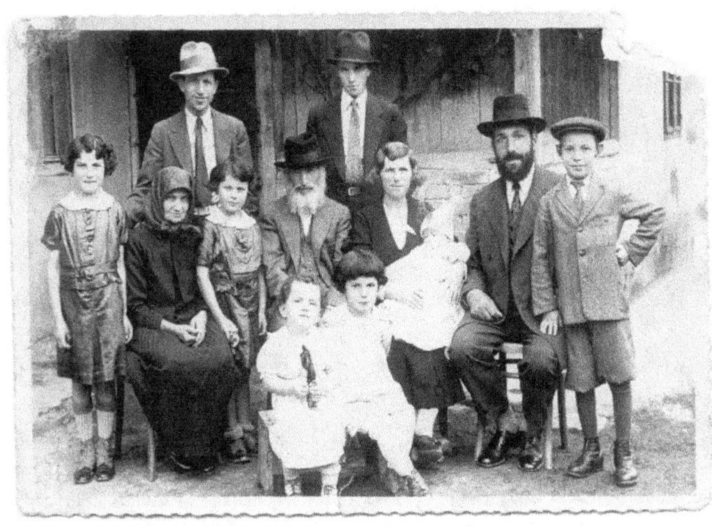

From the viewers' point of view, in the back row left is Joe in the white fedora and Samuel Elias Roth in the black fedora.

Middle Row - from left to right from the viewer's point of view is Roza Chaimovicsova Rothova wearing the scarf, Bernard Roth with the white beard, Berta Rothova Sichermanova with the baby in the lap, and Martin Sicherman with the black beard and black fedora.

Joe had the picture taken by a photographer from Michalovce in 1936. That picture has been studied, and each child and adult has been identified. Samuel Elias, Joe's nephew, is in the back row with the black fedora. Joe Roth is the one with the white fedora. The children are now identified due to the transport list.

Joe tried; he had pluck, and they said no, they did not want to leave. Being resilient in making a decision is not always easy since these people had descendants for 100 years in Vysna Jablonka.

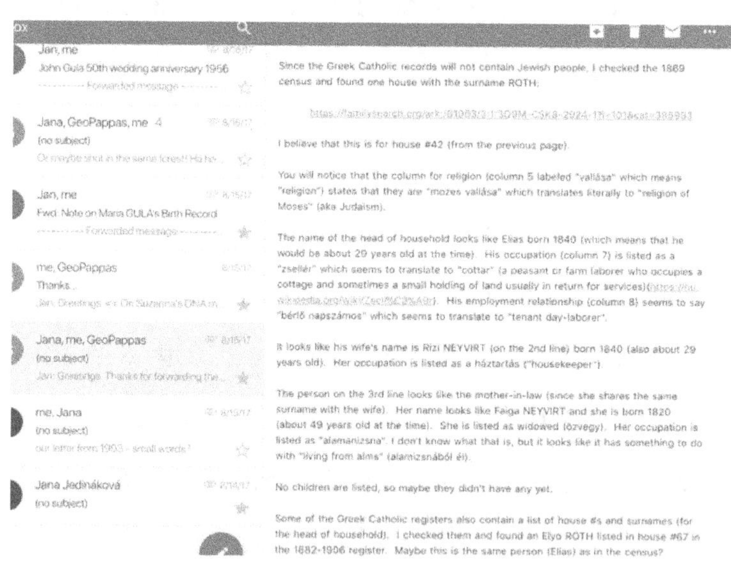

Since the Greek Catholic records will not contain Jewish people, I checked the 1869 census and found one house with the surname ROTH:

https://familysearch.org/ark:/61903/3:1:309M-CSK8-2924-17?i=101&cat=388993

I believe that this is for house #42 (from the previous page).

You will notice that the column for religion (column 5 labeled "vallása" which means "religion") states that they are "mozes vallása" which translates literally to "religion of Moses" (aka Judaism).

The name of the head of household looks like Elias born 1840 (which means that he would be about 29 years old at the time). His occupation (column 7) is listed as a "zsellér" which seems to translate to "cottar" (a peasant or farm laborer who occupies a cottage and sometimes a small holding of land usually in return for services)(https://en.wikipedia.org/wiki/Zsell%C3%A9r). His employment relationship (column 8) seems to say "bérlő napszámos" which seems to translate to "tenant day-laborer".

It looks like his wife's name is Rizi NEYVIRT (on the 2nd line) born 1840 (also about 29 years old). Her occupation is listed as a háztartás ("housekeeper").

The person on the 3rd line looks like the mother-in-law (since she shares the same surname with the wife). Her name looks like Faiga NEYVIRT and she is born 1820 (about 49 years old at the time). She is listed as widowed (özvegy). Her occupation is listed as "alamanizsna". I don't know what that is, but it looks like it has something to do with "living from alms" (alamizsnából él).

No children are listed, so maybe they didn't have any yet.

Some of the Greek Catholic registers also contain a list of house #s and surnames (for the head of household). I checked them and found an Elyo ROTH listed in house #67 in the 1882-1906 register. Maybe this is the same person (Elias) as in the census?

The ancestors of the Roths, as in Bernard's father born in 1840, is what the above document states, were in Slovakia for more than 100 years.

Elias lived in Vysna Jablonka. Chaimovics, Gunczenbergers, and Moskovics had been in Slovakia for 100 to 200 years.

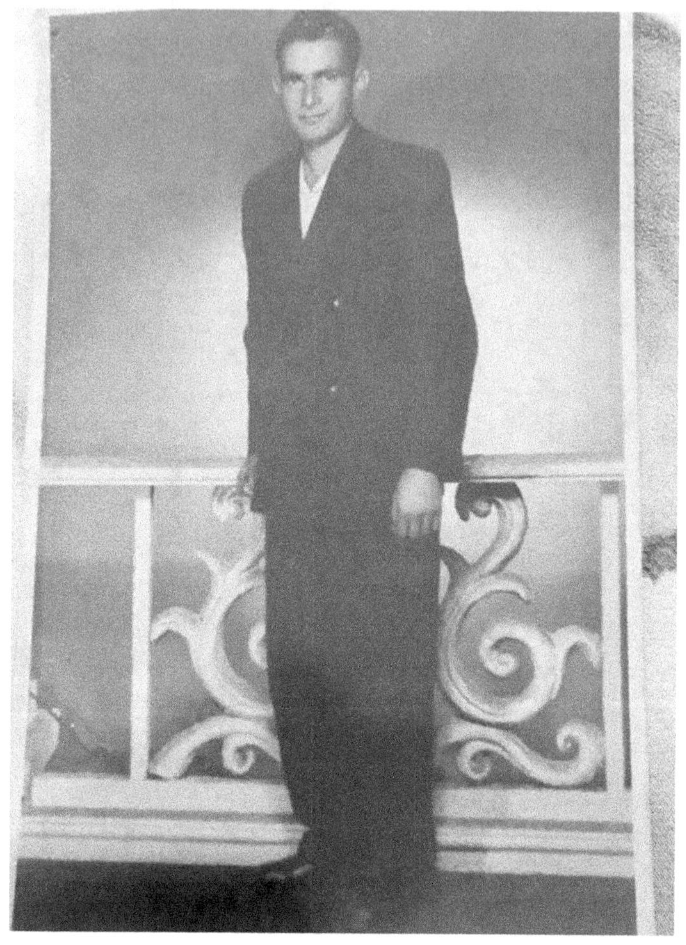

Alex Roth, Sr. is formerly known as Samuel
Elias Roth. Now Samuel Elias Roth, in 1947,
relocated to Teplice, Czech Republic, and he became
a building engineer. He might have changed his
name to honor his Aunt Berta's last baby born in
1942, who had been named Alex.

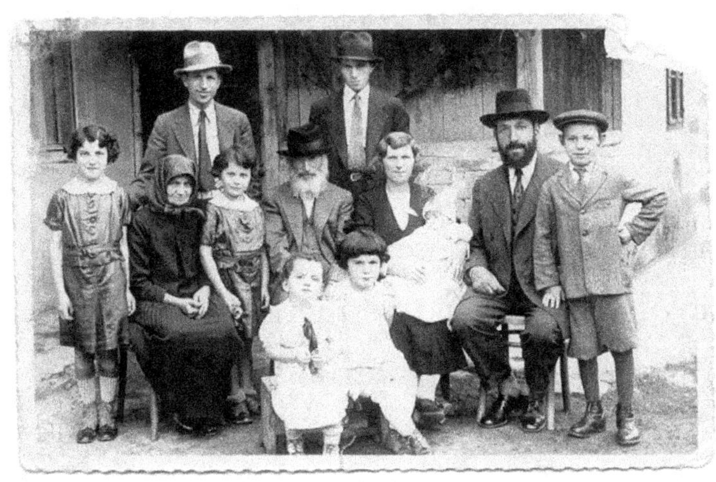

Aunt Berta in the picture has a baby on her lap
and is on the right side, from the viewer's point of
view. Berta is next to the older man with the fedora,
Bernard.

Kata, Jr., the great-great-great granddaughter of
Bernard Roth, said that in later years, Samuel Elias
Roth was saying, "I don't talk about that."

He had married Maria and created 69 people
within this bond. He refused to be interviewed when
a granddaughter requested information about
Auschwitz; in later years, he was happy, but when he

had bad dreams, he would dream and speak in different languages.

This may be why Monro Roth did not find Samuel Elias Roth since his name had been changed to Alex Roth, Sr. and despite a letter being sent to Allentown, Pennsylvania, and Monro filing a Red Cross document searching for Alex, Sr., or rather Samuel Elias Roth in 1947. Alex, Sr. was not found then. In 2023, the grandchild and translator, Sarinka, of Alex, Jr., stated, "In 1948, there was a change of regime. Borders closed. He already had a family here and didn't want to contact anyone." Another answer from the translator, who was the grandchild of Alex Jr. and is in sixth grade in Teplice, Czech Republic, was, "He already had children and wanted to stay here." Something might be lost in the tone of this response, yet it does not negate the American relatives' guilt toward European relatives.

Monro Roth, when asked by his daughter about whether the sergeants had knowledge of the war's atrocities, said that they did not know until the end of the war.

Beatrice Roth, granddaughter of Bernard Roth, who later would become an actress and would write an Off-Broadway play about Helen Roth, was the daughter of Isador who was the son of Bernard. Beatrice also filed a document in which she was looking for Roth relatives after World War II.

According to the translator, in 2022, the great-granddaughter of Samuel Elias, Kata Jr., Samuel Elias, had gotten involved with his wife, Maria.

Samuel Elias Roth was born in 1912, the son of Jakub who died in 1915. Jakub was the son of Bernard Roth.

This Samuel Elias Roth was a miraculous surprise to American relatives in 2019.

Samuel Elias Roth had changed his name to Alex Sr. whose son Alex Jr. matched as a second cousin to the grandchildren of Abe, Isador, and Joe, the sons of Bernard. The great-grandchildren of Bernard Roth were grandchildren of Isador, Abe, and Joe, as Alex is the great-grandson of Bernard Roth. Bernard is the older man with the beard in the picture.

Melinda went to visit in Teplice, Czech Republic, in 2019.

Alex Roth, Jr., who matched with Zuzana, made Melinda realize that Alex was a Chaimovics and part of the Roza Chaimovicsova Rothova and Bernard Roth union. Alex, Jr. is a great-grandchild of the older woman who is Roza Chaimovicsova Rothova and of Bernard Roth, just as the other grandchildren of Joe, Isador, and Abe are.

Roza Chaimovicsova Rothova is a first cousin to Yecheil Chaimovics and also a first cousin to his brother Izrael Chaimovics. The archives later proved this assessment to be correct. And the D.N.A. on

Ancestry corroborated the evidence.

So, one wonders how the laboratory does this. Scientists purify Deoxyribonucleic Acid, which is in every cell of every human, and the order of "beads" is in the same order in every one of the human's cells. This order is now called the genome.

While siblings have 50% identical D.N.A. inside one cell of one sibling with the same order inside another cell of another, whole first cousins have 12.5% identical D.N.A. within each other's cells or about 875 Centimorgans.

One must remember that scientists are looking at D.N.A. for one cell of a human and that the order of "beads" is the same in each cell of one particular human. Second cousins have 6.25% identical D.N.A. with each other's cells or about 446 Centimorgans identical.

Alex and Melinda were discovered through a letter written by Alex's daughter Sona. After the daughter had seen an obituary named Monro Roth on the Internet in 2015, she recognized the name Monro Roth because of the Red Cross document Sona had found in the archives in the Czech Republic.

Alex Roth Jr. was the miracle who was the son of Samuel Elias Roth son of Jakub Roth son of Bernard Roth son of Elias Roth, where Elias was born in 1840, and Jacob Roth who was born before 1840. Alex Jr. was discovered to be a builder of kitchens.

Diagram	
Jacob Roth	
Elias (b.1840-1911)-Naivent,	
Bernard-Chai	Joshua
Jakub- Pachter	Jacob-Lang
Samuel Elias Roth	Saul, Manny

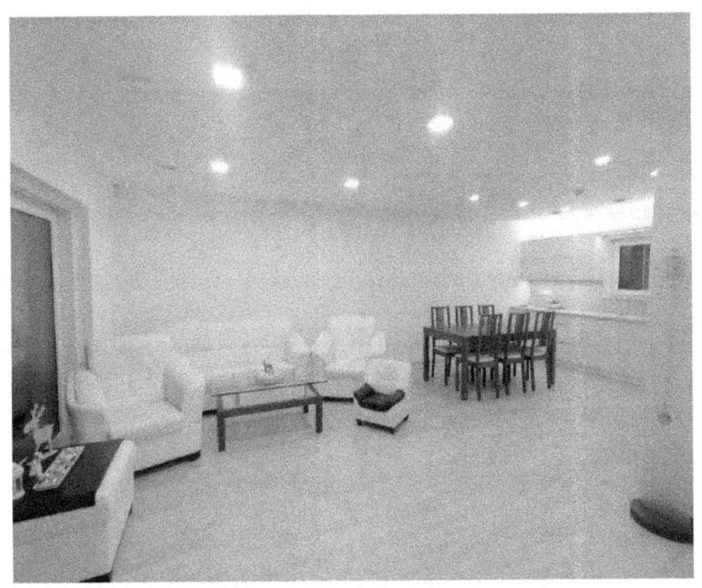

When Alex Jr., in the 1950s, went to school in Teplice, Czech Republic, the others told him they knew he was Jewish because of his eyes. He did not know what "Jewish" was. They also knew that his father had been in Auschwitz. Below, Alex, Jr. is listening as Melinda says the memorial prayer for Alex's grandfather.

Jakub Roth was the grandfather of Alex Jr. Jakub passed away in 1915 before both Jakub's parents Bernard Roth and Rosalie Chaimovicsova Rothova, did.

Diagram	
Bernard	Roth-Roza Chaimovicsova
Isador, Joe, Abe, Jakub (1915), Berta	
	Samuel
	Alex, Jr.
	Sona

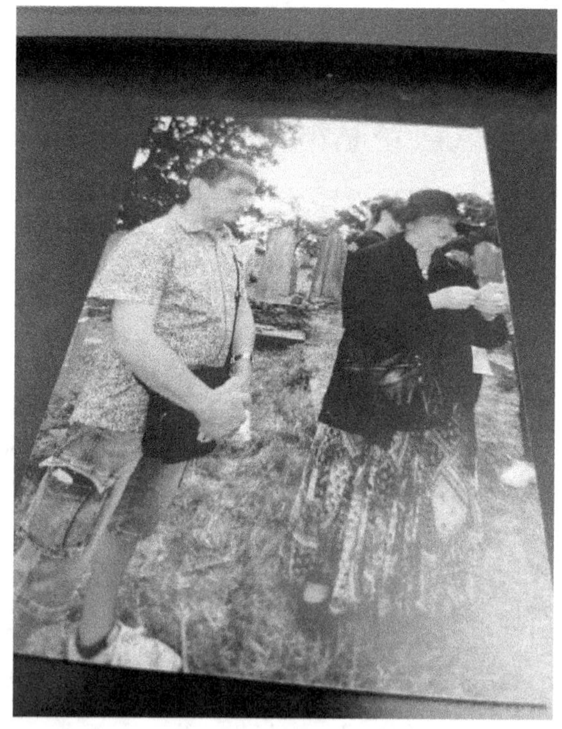

Rosalie Chaimovicsova Rothova, the wife of

Bernard Roth, is a first cousin to Izrael and to Yecheil; all branches of Rosalie's, Yecheil's, and Izrael's descendants match with Zuzana's D.N.A.

This is the story of a woman who discovered her relatives in the Czech Republic in 2019. However, before this happened, a significant amount of work, reflection, and remorse led to this discovery. It is important to share the story of how this woman came to the point of seeking out her family history. As a young girl, she received a letter from a parent that had been sent previously from Europe. Unfortunately, she lost the contents of the letter and did not make any inquiries about her family history at that time. As an adult, she reflected on this missed opportunity and eventually mustered the courage to search for her relatives in 2019.

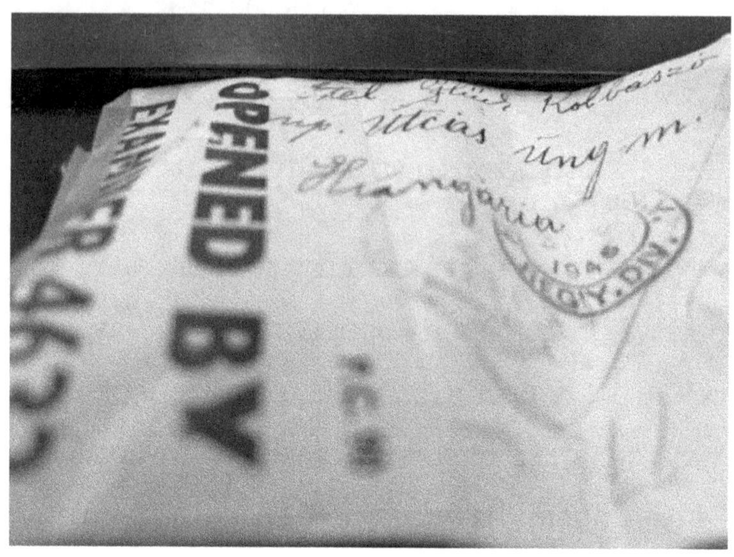

But the woman learned about reflection, remorse, and integrity from her experiences- as when she was in her twenties. The ritual was to travel to New York to visit her maternal grandmother Zelda and great-aunt Bea.

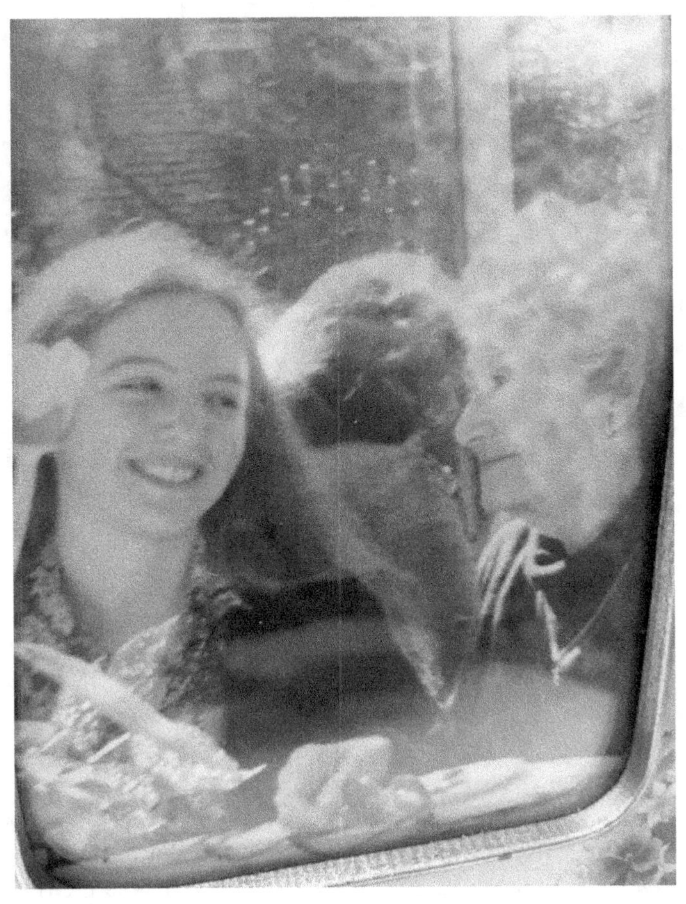

The above picture taken has Zelda Shapiro Gottlieb in it. It was taken in The Twin Towers' Upper Floor Restaurant in 1979.

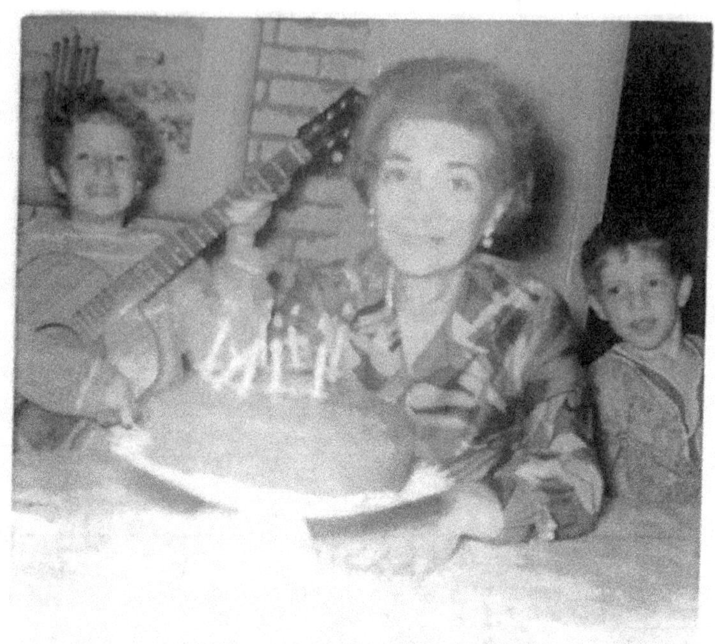

The picture above is of Bertha Shapiro. Bertha
was the wisest person that Mimi Gottlieb Roth,
Zelda's daughter, knew. The woman believed she
had had a visitation from Bertha the day after Bertha
had passed in Mimi's house. After Bertha had gone
to England with her best friend Sylvia, she passed in
her sleep. The woman was wondering what to do
about a dilemma, and Bertha answered her in the
woman's sleep. Sylvia says Bertha would have

"applauded" regarding how she had passed. Bertha or Bea, Zelda's sister, read Russian and English literature and inspired Melinda to read this genre. Bertha had wisdom and a way with her family members. She lived with Zelda.

Once in her apartment, Bea would spin a yarn about the time of how Zelda was climbing up on a chair after a day's cleaning and cooking. Before this time, in Bea's and Zelda's childhood in Brooklyn, their parents placed pots to look like there was a lot of food, and their toes were misshapen by tight shoes. But both Zelda and Bea had become bookkeepers. And so now, Zelda would begin to dust the shades. Beyond the shades were steep cliffs leading to the Hudson River.

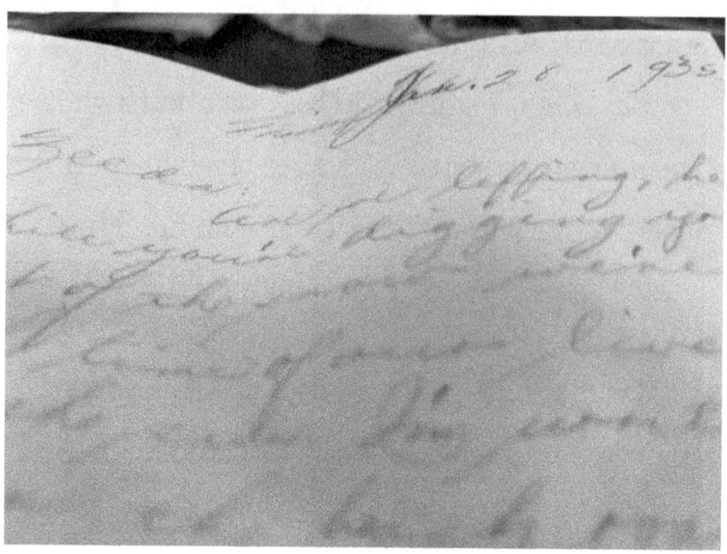

While the woman would hear this story, she would picture Zelda's spry body flinging head over her heels onto the cliffs and onto the river.

Once, the woman asked Zelda why Jimmy Shapiro son of her brother Morris and wife Rose Ruben, lived in Luxembourg.

Zelda answered the woman, "I think there was a custody case."

It was a cocoon there. Before going, the woman would load herself with Godiva for Zelda and

Anthony Trollope novels for Bea. When that nest became too sedentary, Bea, Zelda, and the woman would hike into the Third Reich, Washington Heights' village. The three would walk amidst the wild gardens of Fort Tryon Park and then listen to the smatterings of Germans where the immigrants of World War II were living.

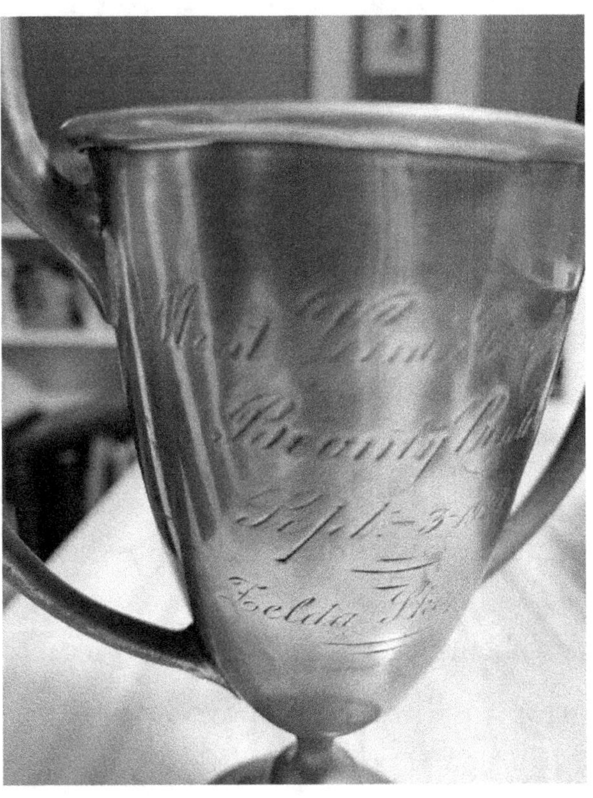

One day, Zelda's probably Prussian fedora-wearing, gray-suited doctor, who on Saturdays strolled the neighborhood, rapped at the door. The woman knew Zelda was feeling honored because Zelda ran to the bathroom to primp.

In the most histrionic and friendly manner, the woman knew how she was ushering him in while vanity had summoned Zelda to a mirror somewhere.

He entered, leaned against the wall, and moaned to the woman what seemed to be a surprising statement, "I should have had a mother, a grandmother for my children. They would have learned to be giving."

It was about at this time Zelda entered, healed from the compliment she had just heard.

Another night, when Zelda wasn't feeling well, the doctor was there again. The room was tinted in a brandy-colored light. He had just finished telling a story of seven sisters, six of whom were too busy going out to charity affairs and were neglecting their other sister, a patient of his.

He glanced over at Bea.

Bea's best friend from their first house, Sylvia Golden, would knit elaborate blankets and paint exquisite copies of master artists.

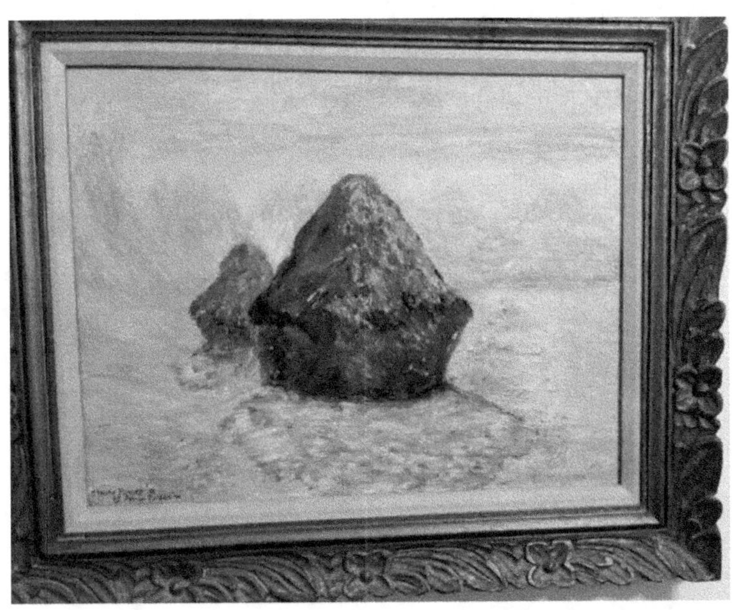

Sylvia once told the woman the story of Morris walking on Bea's washed floor and Bea no longer talking to him, and their mother, Anna Goldwasser

Shapiro, a maybe-cousin to Candidate Goldwater.
Anna told Sylvia to be friends with Bea.

Bea and Sylvia were now working in a public
relations' office and pretending they were not friends,
and they would go to "Nicholas Nickleby," an all-day
Broadway show, and both read Trollope, Austen,
and Dickens. Boss Strauss, who had a relative who
had sunk on the "Titanic" would say, "Anyone who
reads Trollope is a friend of mine."

Bea, born in 1907 of seven siblings of parents
from Warsaw, called this "orphans of the storm."

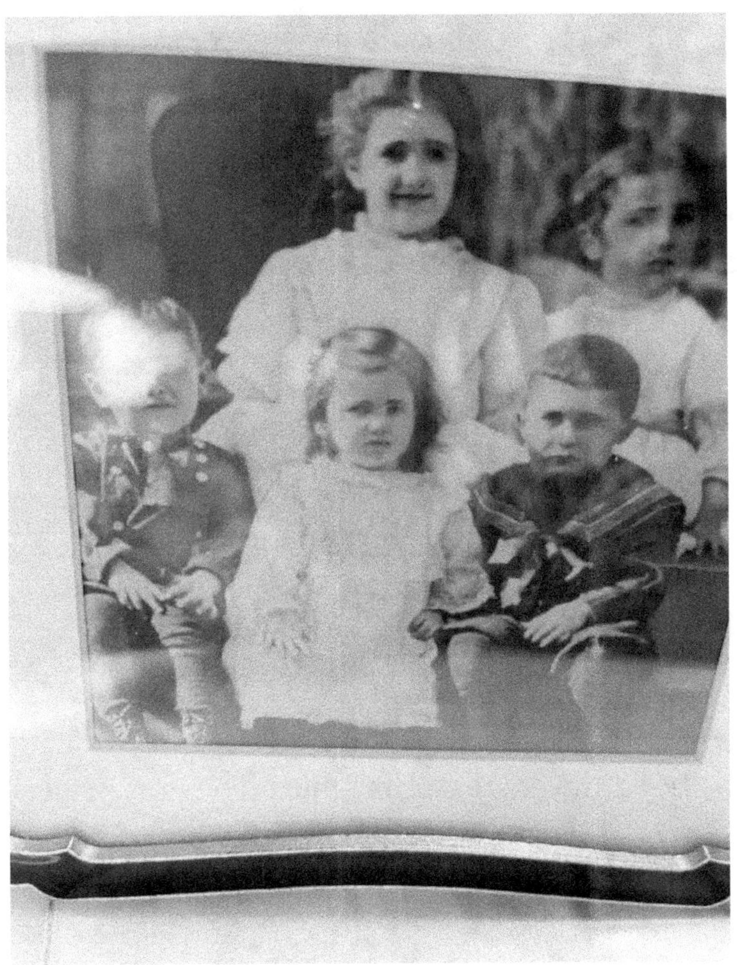

Rose, living in the next apartment house, was another sister to Zelda and Bea.

He explained about Rose, who enjoyed needling him about whether he were a good doctor.

"Sure," he told Zelda and Bea, "she stays long on her visits, but to relieve Bea and let her take a walk, she wouldn't do."

He glanced one more time at Bea furtively. "Bea is a gem," said the woman.

Zelda's emerald eyes began to sparkle.

"Want a drink?" she asked him.

She had just turned eighty-three. The story in the family was that when Rose's doll broke apart, Rose took it upon herself to break Zelda's doll. While the two of them were in their eighties, Rose allegedly kicked Zelda. The woman was ashamed to report this. This happened to Zelda in the shins while in a taxi because Rose believed that Zelda had purposely kicked her.

One could never fear since in D.H. Lawrence's "Sons and Lovers," Writer Lawrence pens that there is an inborn hatred between siblings. On the other side of the woman's family, one Aunt Lucille had broken the doll of another Aunt Shirley, also because a doll, too, had been broken. To quote Lady Colin Campbell, "Oh dear, oh dear, oh dear."

Could the reason some siblings repel each other also be because they share 50% identical D.N.A.? Maybe identical D.N.A. could lead to a blurring of boundaries, a sense of expectation, and worry for the other that could turn into resentment.

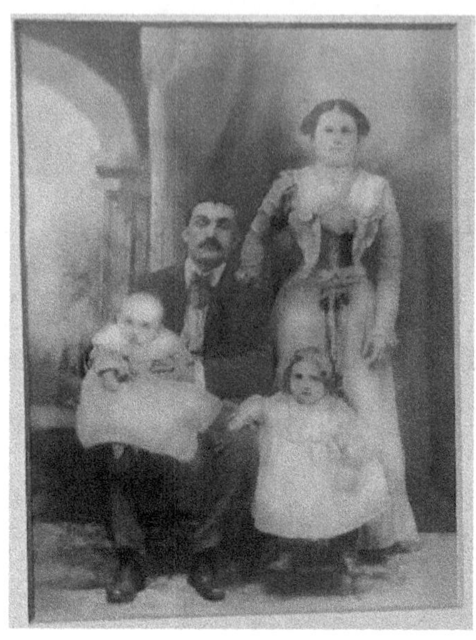

The picture above was taken in 1900 and had
Max Shapiro and Anna Goldwasser Shapiro in the
first upper row from the viewer's point of view, and
in the lower row Rose from the left, and then Zelda.

Well, maybe Rose could empathize with Zelda's
tired and crinkled face, which still retained its beauty
with Grecian-like features. Later on in life, Zelda's
likeness was sketched on a New York bus, and she
was told she had Grecian features.

Zelda, having herself experienced the exhaustion

of standing for long hours while working at Russicks'
department store, still had that beauty. However,
despite all these years, Rose still insisted on claiming
the trophy.

It really had been meant for Zelda. The trophy
stood on Zelda's bookshelf. It had some description
about her and the date 1921 on it.

Soon after spending time with Zelda, the
woman went to Heidelberg to work on assisting in
recombinant D.N.A. as a technician. The choice of
her friend and others subsequently, the woman
would look back later and think of Robin Dunbar's
"Grooming, Gossip, and Evolution of Language,"
published by Harvard Press, of "A Theory of Mind"
where "one can understand what another
individual's thinking" and "would ascribe beliefs,
desires, fears and hopes to someone else," on page
83 and on page 189 Writer Dunbar says that
Marion Petrie "has shown that peahens selectively
prefer peacocks with the largest number of eyespots

on their tails." So, the woman perhaps had deliberately chosen this person. She and her friend went to a small temple for the High Holidays. There was a man there who had been in Auschwitz who beseeched the woman and friend to come back each week.

The hallway was noisy with gaudily-dressed women.

Light came through this plain room in twilight slants while the woman, the gentleman's friend, and a colleague, most likely competing, withstood the long-standing of the last prayer.

At sundown, the congregants ate upstairs. The man from Auschwitz who had been a prisoner drank Schnapps while one teenager with his mother told the woman how he had grown up in a Catholic nunnery.

Sometimes, he whispered to the women and friends he wished he "had never known Germany."

When the woman and the friend returned to the laboratory where they worked, the three who attended this service felt like the other laboratory workers were looking at them.

She guessed that someone must have said something that was odd or painful to these workers in their forties.

Before going to Heidelberg, while being with her grandmother, there always seemed to be company around Zelda; her doctor was regaling her with the letter he had written about the Catholic hospital, which would be closed in Washington Heights. Later, another doctor, Mel Ferrer's brother, said that Zelda had been sicker than others and had never complained. Now, he had been contacted and expressed surprise that she was alive.

Dr. Heller, Zelda's visitor, became more infuriated as he read bits of his letter about the Afghanis he grew up with and said they could live on a fig a day. He shared about his stay in concentration camps and told her he was not convinced that Zelda was so sick.

The woman had promised Zelda she would come home from Heidelberg in the year 1979.

She went to the High Holiday services of about sixty people in Heidelberg. She recalled there was a burly man in his sixties who was praying in sing-song moans and bending to and fro on top of his sneakers.

A scientist working in Heidelberg wondered about the man's sneakers. Weren't they leather? Would he wear them if he were as religious-minded as he said?

Some days passed. Dorte, a Danish scientist, called the friends aside, and they went to drink spirits at 4:00 P.M. in the laboratory's cafeteria.

There, Dorte told her friends her childhood

stories of how her father would place his ear onto the radio set, tuned to the illegal BBC channel in Nazi-held Denmark.

Dorte then said, "I learned that languages were very important." "After the war," she said, "children were in cellars gobbling potatoes hungrily like animals, and one scientist who was half-Jewish received a letter to report to a work camp." He said he "thought it was a dream." His friends "were standing in the streets in new uniforms jovially hitting their necks and explaining what would happen" if they "reported."

Dorte continued her story:

The scientist never went to the camp. He hid in the woods and survived.

Then the woman walked into an antique store in downtown Heidelberg, and there was a menorah, and she was being called Madchen by the saleswoman.

The others had come to work on recombinant D.N.A. - these others and the woman witnessed this world of blue vapor of the Kaiserstuhl Mountains that still rise above the flora of Heidelberg.

There were lush trees in Heidelberg's mountains, along with what she believed in 1979 to be ghosts moaning and bending their boughs. She and her friends were in an autobus climbing these mountains toward where they went to work at a biochemistry laboratory.

They walked through mountainous passages during the holiday.

One of the friends wished to celebrate the High Holidays while he would be adhering to the religion. He didn't turn his lights on that weekend. They stayed till late evening.

Walking through those mountains reminded the woman of her grandmother and the man the grandmother loved - her Prussian doctor.

She wanted to go to Philadelphia then; her friend was going to graduate school in California. He said he didn't want to have to teach her how to cook. She relocated to a high-rise building in Center City and began a teaching certification program.

Raymond was a colleague where the woman worked.

He had almond-shaped eyes that made him appear handsome, with a soupcon of Spaniard sprinkled with Native American and a dab of African. She always said he could talk to a pauper by saying, "I got this." Or soothe kings while guarding Philadelphia places.

Reasoning helped Raymond now. Both the woman and Raymond worked together as he would spin his stories. Succor saved him too, he said, as parole guys saw his excreting.

He talked about how he had gotten into trouble.

"I never robbed nobody," he once said. That reminded the woman of when she had a student in Philadelphia schools who said, "She not no fighting girl."

His motto regarding the past days was always, "Act on instinct."

"Guys go with gut feelings," Raymond said.

Therein lay the quandary.

Like some Philadelphians, childhood Raymond sprinted from roof to roof. Over three-floor houses dubbed Trinities, he would fly.

Teenage Raymond was going along with instinct thing when he lived and worked there. The boss in Orthodox garb in Brooklyn would demand that Raymond break windows. The boss would mend them and then make money. Raymond cashed in.

Later on in life, remorse kicked in like a throbbing wound while he was spinning stories and making minimum wage. One tale was about a coworker who said he did not date his own kind.

"Really," said another coworker, "Well, it takes one to know one," she shot back. Raymond tittered, so unfamiliar with that saying.

Yes, Raymond was a coworker. He had been on the wrong side of the crib for a time. Now, he was making his life better.

One night, he scored a sale in Philadelphia in his other life. Then he got locked up. He said he always went by premonitions, but not that night though.

Well, that time was when he got caught. Thirty thousand bucks had been taken off him by a cop. He said, "People didn't file no papers when stereos get smashed." something that had happened where he now worked, "Nah, you take his, he takes yours," he said.

But his broken-hearted mother, who cleaned

houses, and stepfather, whom Raymond never really liked, both cried when Raymond got locked up. The stepfather was now a Coworker too. He said Raymond had made one right decision of not having kids.

His stepfather was the one who visited him for four years while he was in the "clink." Raymond said he learned who came to see him when chips were down and who didn't.

In jail, a female guard tornado-tossed things while looking. Raymond had Street Smarts about Women. He stayed away from fists for the first time as he wrote what happened on paper. Then, he gave the paper to higher-ups.

Before that moment, he said, all was fisticuffs and grabbing drugs off dealers from Badlands.

Now, one important thing at that moment was paper and pen, and Raymond said he learned that a pen was mightier than a fist.

Raymond's reflection or thinking about stuff he was about to do now came into play. And he never knew that knowing two languages was a badge and not a shame until his Coworker pointed it out.

Raymond's ex-girl called, cried, and said she didn't have cash for lights to be on.

She was the one, he told, about how his ex-girl made his fifty-eight hats-dashing, dapper, derbies, jockeys, and other jaunty caps disappear. It's no wonder a professor once warned an inner-city teacher, "Never touch a guy's hat."

'Cause it sure was a "Curious George" yarn there in Raymond's Inner City. "Does anyone still wear a hat?" Stephen Sondheim's crooners crooned.

Now Raymond was a coworker, and someone at work said, "There are people in places where men are few and money rare. And heroes with windfalls step up and save the day."

So, he paid his ex-girl's bill, and the lights came on.

There was a woman who spoke to his coworker. She said, "He was a different guy," in the 'hood, he had gotten boiling mad . . . despite his charm at work. She spoke about rage and a bat.

Meanwhile, he told his coworker about the woman's line she gave to him of "Knocking off socks." The coworker was discovering a scary side to him too.

There are second acts in life.

One should not let anyone tell otherwise.

Raymond's Coworker became a teacher in threadbare and drug-torn Kensington, named after posh English Kensington. One woman, when hearing a student at a community college after hearing the English- accented student say he was from Kensington, she piped up in Philadelphia that she too was from Kensington. That guy was told that could have been a teachable moment. Instead, he left there. Now, the student's name was read in America's Kensington: Raymond with the tag Junior. He was queried about whether his father had worked at a high-end building.

So now the son was sitting in class.

Raymond's brother was hauling a truck, now wearily tramping in for a teacher's meeting. He had wiped off his parents' row home's mortgage with new pay. He did that by driving a truck with a newly gotten license, all done in a gussied-up neighborhood.

The coworker was happy this was happening. Raymond's brother claimed to have "never seen people running in his parts except from cops." Instead, in the high end, twentysomethings were running carefully cultivating bodies. Now Raymond's brother was on hand to tell Raymond, Jr. about getting religion and going to school while the actual

Raymond was once again in the "hole." He had bit someone's ear this time, his baby mamma's guy, and now, Raymond was attending a violence group.

Meanwhile, the coworker bumped into Raymond in Kensington when his wife was pregnant with baby number two. Coworker visited his Trinity Row home with a red Oriental rug splashed on wooden parquet floors. That rug looked real good in there that at work had been given to him.

Raymond said baby one used to peer out the window while waiting for Raymond to come home.

Time passed. Five babies later, Raymond called the coworker. They walked along South Street to "Tritone," dubbed after a devil's three-pitch fork. Rick, the bartender who never watched television and only read books, locked his gaze on Raymond.

Raymond's eyes were pinched into tiny radii back then.

Another time, Raymond walked into Kensington Park with the coworker after dropping his son off at school. Raymond had met the mother of his children, a simple woman. She baked and cooked, he said. She was no longer in the mountains of Puerto Rico.

She could only communicate in Spanish.

Now, five children later, he was coming to his son's school. Soon after, the mother of his son took a pill for mania, went to his workplace, and became hysterical.

Consequently, the marriage unraveled. . .that and the biting of the ear. There was something about another guy, an ear bitten, and an anger management program in jail. He explained that to the Coworker.

Now, in the year 2020, the Coworker thought of Raymond jumping roofs and how he said he never thought he'd live this long. 'Cause once again, with the American President gesticulating on television after he had gotten better from a Virus, it felt like Icarus going up to the sun with a Chariot and a Fatal Flaw.

The coworker was reminded of Raymond jumping roofs.

Surely, the President would now show some learning that would knock into his head.

After all, the President now called himself Superman.

People believed him as he offered his drug cocktail to people as the virus continued to be exponential and airborne.

But afterward, he kept going out into arenas.

Was there still no reflection in this president's psychological makeup? The president was still a performer. He soothed and appeared to make anything possible. Maybe he was sympathetic since he wore his heart on his sleeve.

In youth, there were things that an older guy thought over his life he would regret. Hyperactive President in childhood hit a toddler.

Raymond's Coworker did acts by instinct too. When a neighbor told her to drop the eggs, she brought a bird's nest down in childhood.

Parents Mimi and Monro had told her that night, "Would you jump off a building if someone told you to do that?" That action haunted the Coworker.

Sometime later, the woman turned sixteen. She was given gads of paperwork to canvas a neighborhood. She couldn't handle the running around. She didn't follow through and let the paperwork get thrown out. That was guilt.

Next, her teenage-self worked at an amusement park. She was being trained. She almost missed buckling them in. The supervisor belted them in.

Here, she was grateful for an eternity.

Reflection, like some kind of fine wine, had redefined those times.

Reflection made the coworker, the Guard Raymond, and, well, maybe the President, see a way.

Back in childhood, with these three, maybe the young needed to be watched because the adults weren't always there. With age came remorse but also forgiveness.

Who doesn't tell the story of one's life and

relearn new ways?

Was it possible that the President was appealing to people not for greater good but for attention?

Maybe he would find another way if he didn't win the election rather than continue gathering people in arenas. But people surely would preserve The Union and Appeal for the Greater Good. So, the Denizens voted in 2020.

Before that, that woman had restarted out at 17 years of age with the gig "Life and Romantic Lives" and "Living Life with Purpose," so her intention was never to hurt, and she had chosen the scientist.

After six years of suffering, a sibling passed at the age when she was seventeen. She struck a deal with God to be good and wanted to find a job that required curing the illness that took her sibling. She enrolled in a public institution and began studying biology. She recalls staring up at the stars splotched throughout the sky like dazzling white coverlets. She had never seen stars fill a sky so solidly before in that little town, so she made her pact.

After three years of studying, it was now the beginning of summer. She accompanied her mother, Mimi, to a New York airport. They were waiting for the other sibling to come home.

She said to her mother, "Let's play tribal geography."

They looked around and searched for people from their little town. The mother found two sisters and struck up a conversation.

And sweet they were.

She still remembers what she was wearing. She had a jean jumper on. She was being charming in a newly self-possessing way.

One sister said she wanted to fix her up with her son. As soon as she mentioned his name, she knew him from the science fair and Harvard admittance as a sophomore and media coverage from that little town.

That week, he called, and she went out in her little town. The first date was in the "Traylor Hotel," where there was a restaurant.

The woman walked there. He walked there. Red light, symbolically that is, maybe, telling her about his brother, he said in a not-so-kind way, "Do you want to meet him?"

Still, she persevered at 21 years of age. He ordered wine and tasted the wine first.

She had never seen that.

He quoted a song and said he did not like talking about science with non-scientific people.

On another date, he took her to the New York opera. He said he had heard about her father and the furniture business. It had been in trouble.

So, they sat in Paley's Park and were surrounded by cascades of water; she answered that she had heard about his father's amours. She was sad as his eyes welled up, but she wanted him to know how much it hurt her that he brought up her father's bankruptcy in business.

It was a new experience for her. The next day, he cooked what was a gourmet meal. Her parents had now gone away to England. This man was now stating rules to her. He was going to another country. He would be working in science. But he would not be there for her when he would return in one year unless she would go with him.

One humiliation occurred while the father was jostling with the German shepherd. "Not in front of an innocent woman," said the father to the dog. Only…the father said another word.

Suffice it to say she went without listening to signals, instinct, or marriage. She went with him after finishing a Bachelor's in Science a year later. She remembers her father saying, "You're not going there without marriage, are you?"

But the lack of her use of conventions was not the problem because he fit into her credo of living life with purpose by trying to find scientific cures.

She did not know.

Erich Fromm says in "The Art of Loving" that one chooses to love and does not fall in love. She had decided, but disturbing things continued to occur. Yes, she was still innocent, to not be able to handle little humiliating remarks in public, just the way his father would talk to his mother.

She did not want to answer those remarks in kind nor seem like a bickering couple. That is what she told her father when he picked them up at the New York airport after one year was over.

The friend was bossing her father onto a byway.

Her father said he appreciated she did not want to act like a bickering couple.

But during that past year, while in Denmark, a Lebanese saleswoman selling a porcelain figure of what was called "Married Couple" after hearing his remarks, said to him, "Treat her kindly. We are all tourists on this earth."

Recently, she found that sculpture "The Married Couple" is missing from her parents' house. Did the boyfriend take it?

He had gone with her to her great uncle Morris's and great aunt Rose's house, who were prominent in politics. . .below is Eleanor Roosevelt with Rose Ruben Shapiro-

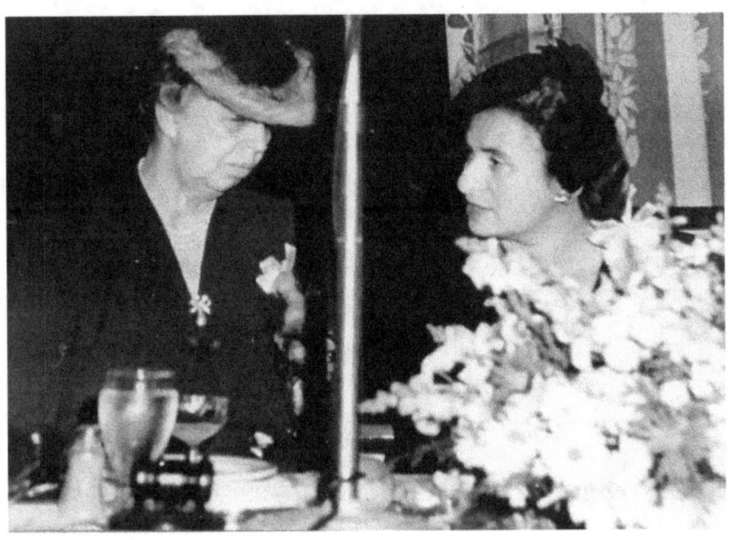

...when her mother gave Uncle Morris a statue, Uncle said, "That's for dead people," and the spirited mother said, "Did you hear that?"

In front of the boyfriend, she had taken her statue home. Did the "boyfriend" model the mother's behavior? She did remember that when she was back home, her boyfriend asked to see the statue, and her mother said, "Want it back?"

His mother had come to visit while they were in Europe. He had traveled and left his mother for approximately one hour while in Europe, and when he wanted to drive up a mountain, the mother was upset in a subdued manner.

He had told the woman later that the woman's mother's behavior with the uncle was OK and acceptable. You see the pattern, dear reader?

The woman was young, dumb, and naïve, afraid of making any decision, and was slowly ceding power.

While she and her friend had gone to the Scandinavian countries that past year, she was hiking and saw a redheaded boy amidst a blue expanse of ocean. She knew she was in rapture when the boy reminded her of someone.

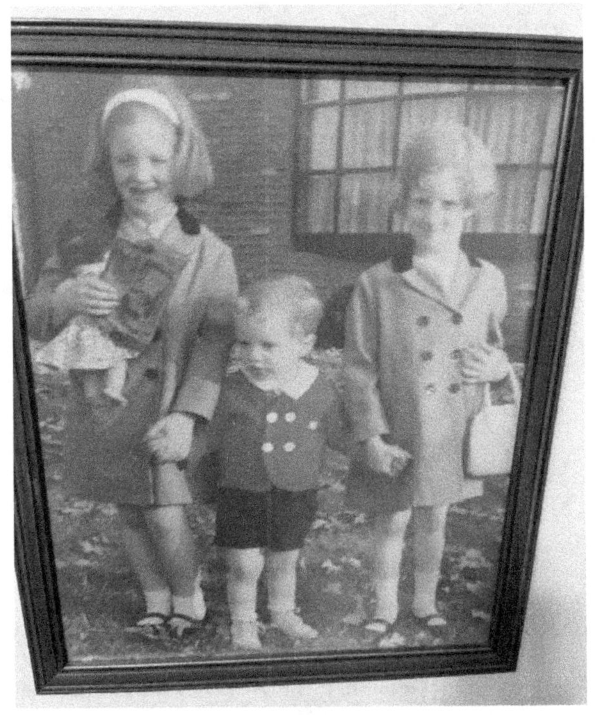

He asked then what was the matter.

Always, their conversational pairs were flouted.

The friend had gone to Norway because he had a course to take in recombinant D.N.A., and now, at the end of his course, there was a huge, steep escalator in a subway in Denmark. He wanted her to go down the escalator with two suitcases, one suitcase in each hand, one of which was his; she could not.

She worked in a laboratory in Germany and as a waitress for the American Army at a non-commissioned officers' club. They told her that she could not miss the holiday of New Year, so she had to wait to go to Norway and thus traveled alone.

The friend had already gone to Norway.

On the train to Norway solo from Germany, the Yugoslav. . .yes, it was when that country was still united, a Yugoslav sat next to her with no one else in the car. He talked and seemed to get physically closer; the train director saw this and had her removed.

Then, on the train, a man spoke in German to

her about how he feared his son was going to the Israeli war. His eyes turned red as he narrated the story.

Next, a Swedish woman told her story about how when Swedish women would go to Italy, they would come back with bellies full because Swedish men weren't forward enough.

"Salty dogs," which meant sailors, but they were not aggressive, she said, unlike the Italians, and punctuated her speech with the big heaping breaths Swedes used for the word "Yes." She had thought that something was wrong in a respiratory way until she saw that all the Swedes were doing this breathy "Ya."

When she finished this trip by herself to get to Norway, which took three days, to meet the friend, she blurted out in English to the couple that she had been talking in German to, "I don't know where to go."

They were baffled.

Regardless, the friend met her at the Tromso station, one of the most exotic places she had ever seen and one of the most exquisite, with fjords of water pouring down upon mountains.

Later on, when she was in the subway with him at the end of this trip, she was facing the steep escalator, and he insisted that she go down with a suitcase in each hand. The berating would have continued, but…

…a very tall, African-descent Danish employee approached her; he said he would take her on the elevator.

The man told her that going down that escalator would have been dangerous. She was too young and dumb and withdrawn, to acknowledge her gratitude to the subway employee.

Despite all of that, she was still giving the

Harvard graduate a pass.

While on a hike in Norway, she was gazing at the sea- such beauty- when she saw the redheaded boy swimming and thought she was seeing a visitation of the lost sibling.

He inquired as to what was different. She remained silent. Previously, on a trip with him to the Lofoten Islands of Norway the path had a mountainous rising of one hundred and eighty degrees up and the other side dangerously descending to the sea.

The friend was hiking ahead of her in Tromso, above the Arctic Circle, and he was seemingly irritated by her slowness and cries.

The next day, a girl on the hike told her how annoyed he was with her and that the girl had had a friend like that.

Next, the friend wanted to go up higher on a

mountain in Tromso to see the Native Norwegians, the Lapps.

One girl approached her in that shelter and asked in Norwegian, "Are you Norsk?" Nor did she know how to greet his colleagues that evening, and he then showed her a letter to his mother about how he would marry the woman after she had been inflicted with a mosquito-bitten body from waiting for him at the shelter.

Then, in Sweden, a woman began to speak to her friend while walking on stones by the shore. She was informing him that a developmentally challenged young girl had blurted out, "You tourists only come with good weather." He had revealed his life plans to the Swedish woman, and his plans did not seem to include the woman.

She turned to the other woman, and the other woman remarked portentously to the woman, "You better find yourself something to do in life."

Then, she began craving an apple in Norway after she had heard that fruit was not grown there. Caving in, she bought an apple for a dollar.

She must have been glaring because the salesman asked what was wrong. Yet again, she was too young, dumb, and withdrawn to be able to explain with compassion that the price was the shock and not self-aware enough to express her gratitude for his concern.

The older people were hiking up mountains; their idea of a good time was a cabin without electricity, the friend said.

One year after living in the other country, he told her he needed to go to graduate school, and he did not want to have to teach her how to cook.

Her great aunt Bea, the angel on her shoulder, said, "I guess it kind of eliminates the rat race to have him as a friend."

That remark was sort of a shock to her, too.

After endless struggles with new careers, she found a living and avocations, yet she has not had the mundane intimacy since. Still, romance and an odyssey of life continued.

One of the statements her friend came up with was that he did not want to teach her how to cook. Now she had proof of his lack of liking the human being because he had just been divorced from his present wife, who had lost her job in hospital administration. Well, perhaps the woman had a tad of schadenfreude.

He had a way of making someone feel bad when the chips were down. He did not know how to love, but perhaps she was looking at accomplishments and overlooking his public humiliation of people; maybe she did not know how to love either.

Well, the second way was a radio talk host; she

had written a letter in calligraphy while she was living in a dangerous area. He called her, and after six months, he lost his job and said he would have to move.

The third one, she wrote a letter to. . .he had been pistol-whipped in Vietnam and wrote an account of that in the newspaper.

One should not blame her, dear reader; she was an inner-city teacher with perfect attendance. She was taking buses and trains in Philadelphia, Pennsylvania. It had not occurred to her that one could sit in a bar and get a drink and talk and play the jukebox.

An epistolary relationship began with her epistles to him, which she illustrated; she knew him rather "metaphorically" and saw him for eight years.

His final way of leaving was that he needed to travel to China to write because the man died from the cannon rolling on him, tragically, in Tiananmen Square. He then told her to find a man who would "appreciate all" she "has to give."

Now that she was a "lady," it made her realize she could leave someone, so she did. She went out with another for six months. He took drugs. She never did. Going out with him was one mistake.

She made one mistake: she chose a guy with several degrees after her first one. She decided she had to try to date. This new guy had a degree in philosophy from an Ivy League school, a law degree, and had attended the beginning of a writer's program from an Ivy League school. He had a perfect score on the S.A.T., he said.

She met him at a bar next door to her building; she would have never thought of going into the bar, but her older neighbor talked her into it then.

This new guy would read books and "New Yorker" magazines all day in a tavern. That was the first warning signal.

His father was a doctor, so she questioned whether she should go out with him because he seemed to do nothing. She decided to go out with him. This time, she would try to help someone else and maybe help make his life better. She went out with him for several months.

After that first meeting, he read and read books; she found out that he smoked marijuana all day and tried muscle relaxers.

He compared himself to Coleridge, an opium-addicted poet. He once said he was nothing but a drug addict, but she couldn't believe that. She thought he was being dramatic. She learned that one must believe when someone tells what he is.

He also told her how he used to go to the professor's office at Columbia and argue. His theory was to argue until either the professor a) changed the grade or b) the professor kicked him out of the office.

She told him, "Well, can't you take that energy and apply that to a job?"

He responded that he had "a problem..."

Next, his maid was sitting in the dark as if she could not turn on the lights; even he felt she should turn on the lights. But this was his style of luxury of having a cleaning woman without himself having or seeking a job.

Then, after he had moved into a posh apartment, paid for by his father, she went over there and looked out at the magnificent South Philadelphian view. He began telling a story about how he had been arguing with a girlfriend.

The police had told him to stop; he explained to the woman and said he had answered back defiantly to the police. The police then got out of the car. She said, "Well, you shouldn't have disobeyed the police." Suddenly, he became subtly moody.

Did she mention that he had a bookcase that covered all the walls? And on that wall, he had Bacchus or Dionysus, the god of wine and substances. He had the god of Bacchus on his wall poster.

His English friend told her later that he had usually gathered women in the park but was happy with her. He said he liked people who did not do drugs, yet she wasn't listening carefully because now she had gone out.

She was struggling with teaching and several jobs. One should be clear: she did not have two cents to rub together, and the rent was a problem. She did not get money from anyone nor him, thankfully.

But then he advised her when she was too scared to go to her job as an inner-city teacher. He said, "Just get there." That piece of advice she heeded for the rest of her life.

He was insistent about going out. In fact, for the

first and last time, he pressured and threatened her and hurled items outside his door.

When she looked at a notebook of his, which she was wrong for doing that herself, the Ivy Leaguer, an unemployed person, had Monday to call his apparent dealer, Tuesday to call a certain girl, Wednesday to call another girl, and so on, one thing per day and nothing else on that page whereas another person would have filled notes out about job hunting.

One time, he came with her to visit a writer, her great uncle Morris' son-in-law, Jerry. There, he kept going to the men's room. Her great-aunt Bea noticed and told her later he kept going to the men's room. She hadn't noticed. Then, at his father's funeral, his sister resentfully called him "a drug addict."

Yes, he was a diabetic type II, "Not that there was anything wrong with that," credit to Jerry Seinfeld, but she found out.

Later, when she ended this, she learned of his drug taking from an older couple whom he had befriended from "Elan," a nightclub. That man was so charming that he had friends there called "Knights of the Round Table."

That older man never had to pay for a drink at "Elan." This Ivy League guy had stolen medicine from this older man's cabinet, as the older man later told the woman.

He didn't want her to talk to others, so when a friend came from college to visit, and she walked the friend back to his car, Ivy Leaguer was angry. She felt like she was being monitored and watched all the time.

She began to want to talk to anyone, for instance, taxi drivers, servers, and anyone who had a job and was doing something.

Her father had a conference in the city where she lived. This guy called her apartment and was slurring his words to her father. She explained to her father that he took muscle relaxers.

Her father, who worked at a community college, told her he worked with students who have jobs, responsibilities, and school, and they don't do that. Her father said, "You mean he reads books in the middle of the afternoon?"

She then spoke to the Ivy League guy over the telephone. She ended the conversation by saying, "You can't handle life's problems."

She used to feel in being naïve that when one begins with someone, it is a sin to discontinue, but after the constant harassment of his calling, throwing things, consuming marijuana, and threatening to call the job, little she, who believed that if she committed to something, said, "Get this, it's over." She did not like being like that, but she felt endangered.

This guy would read books all day, use his father's secondary credit card for himself, and go out, and she happily got out of that. She thought it was immoral to get out of something, yet it was better, she finally felt, to be alone than with the wrong person.

One more thing that Dr. Michael King, a psychologist, pointed out was, "The exploiting of undergraduates occurs by men who hang out on campuses."

She then recalled that this guy used to say that he had realized there was a use for psychology and that he should have gone to a psychologist.

Following several months of this, he delivered something embarrassing to the front desk of her building; he pushed her out of his apartment after she had refused something and saw a stranger who came to his apartment to sell something; he went to South Street to try to purchase what she had learned was "an expensive form of marijuana," another person had told her; then she ended it.

She was relieved when she saw him with a woman. That lovely woman went on to write three books with him, and this other woman was relieved to be left alone in terms of just the telephone.

When she began to go out with him, she was 29 years old and struggled even with a college degree, which made her susceptible at that time. That lasted six months.

That is why the woman always tells women and men that a skill with honest money for a job is important. It doesn't matter what that job is -as long as one can get through the day with that and that it is "clean" money. She now felt that one could always read at night as an autodidact.

Every man and woman needs a job, or if a person has income, then a purpose. As Oprah Winfrey said, and the woman finally realized, "First time a victim, second time a fool."

Now, the woman veered in her thinking once

again to the Romantic Route along with the commonsensical way, and she realized, as they say in Philadelphia, Pennsylvania, "Common Sense is not common."

Excuse Number One from the female who had become the lady-he took drugs.

She dated a fifth, who is a writer, and she was busy, and so was he. There were no excuses. It was lovely to quote Robert Redford in "The Way We Were."

And then, finally, she dated the sixth; she met him at a part-time job, and she began to care.

With apologies to Singer and Songwriter Carole King, "Her Life Has Been" like a beautifully stranded necklace of opals, glistening colors — turquoise, pink, white, and black — that life like a necklace brings sparkly hues as in friendships. First, she mentioned her friend Anna Magnani named after the movie, "The Rose Tattoo."

Anna played a part where she was always lachrymose and melancholic. She was mourning a man who had left her, and her chest was tattooed with a red rose. Burt Lancaster played her paramour or attempted paramour. Amidst the muggy climate of New Orleans, in this movie, the actor tried to cheer up Anna Magnani's character, and all she did was discuss her other lover. In the movie, Burt Lancaster drove a fruit truck, and to oblige and cheer her, he got himself a rose tattoo for his chest. Did she cheer up?

Nah, but in real life, her friend Anna had a drink called "Rose with Thorns" while everyone had left the city of Philly for the seashore.

A long time ago, when she and Anna Magnani began to teach, Anna went out with another woman, parked her car, got locked out, climbed over the fence, and got locked up. That plot was in the movie, "The Walk of Shame," so she must have accidentally told that story to the scriptwriter.

Well, tonight, Anna's name of the drink was coincidental to what this story had portrayed her to be. But the Anna Magnani character in the movie, did she cheer up?

Nah, but the friend Anna fell in love with a gentleman who behaved like the rose, or did she behave like the prince in "The Little Prince" by Antoine De Saint- Exupery? In that story, the rose is prickly, but the prince insists on loving the rose. Antoine De Saint- Exupery died in a plane accident in World War II. A poem of his was quoted when a teacher was lost in a flight with astronauts, and all were lost in the air. In his book, "The Little Prince," he stated, "And your friends will be properly astonished to see you laughing as you look up at the sky."

Her friend tried to tell the guy to study when he had been taking illegal pills, and she tried to tell him to quit smoking. He did and became an emergency technician and then a paramedic.

She kept loving him because she said he had the sensibilities to understand her complexity. Yes, he was an "old head," as they say in the non-mainstream dialect of Philadelphia.

She was beautiful. A lot of guys harassed her for this. She spent money on eyebrows, facials, working out, on her son, and on her mother. She continued to love that guy who was overly devoted to his mother, and he claimed he had left her because she "talked about his mother."

She had a difficult job, just like the woman had. She was an inner-city teacher, and now she was finally free for the summer, so she bought herself a dog. The reader may wonder why certain people are masochists. So, when her friend finally could go out, she said she could not because of the dog.

The other beautiful bead on the woman's opal necklace was Michael.

She walked through the lobby of her building decades ago and saw a mechanic working at the desk with red floppy hair who was about six feet tall. She said to the desk clerk, "You have him working for you now."

He seemed like that giant in "Rudolf, The Red Nosed Reindeer," an animated movie so wisely written when the monster hangs the star on the Christmas tree.

Fast forward, she got a job at the desk while she was a substitute teacher with her biology degree. She was there when the electricity went out, the heating went out, and the water stopped.

There were four people stuck in the elevator.

The mechanic who had been recently hired, perhaps through nepotism, asked her what to do, so she called the fire department.

Then in walked burly lumberjack Michael with

his beautiful red beard, and as she screamed, "Four people are stuck in the elevator," he went to the elevator and screamed, "Yo, what floor you on?"

They told him, and he crawled from that floor to the aperture to where the elevator was. One lady, he said, had said, "Get me out; I am a very important person."

She was working with him, and another desk clerk said, "Everything you do is for yourself."

She was offended, so Michael called her in the middle of the night and said, "Never let people get to you." He then confided that he had wanted to be a football player.

That talk may have changed her life. All the older ladies had to have him fix something for them, so he also fixed their things and sometimes their souls.

The woman thought of J.D. Salinger's daughter's biography, where she wrote about climbing a mountain in a posh northeastern American town in the 1960s when almost all of the teachers and students were cruel in her posh private school. As she tried to climb that mountain, one teacher patiently asked her if she were OK, and she never forgot that. In her book, she quoted the beautiful Hebrews 13:2: "Be not forgetful to entertain strangers: for thereby some have entertained angels unaware." That quote reminded the woman of Michael.

One lady he carried from the bed to the bathroom left him an account; he said that he had paid his bills. The third shift in a row, he was reading the bible.

Working with him was a treasure of an experience and reminded her of the story by D.H. Lawrence's "Kangaroo," when they quietly were reading to each other. The joy was that love happened coincidentally in a place she had never planned- in a world she had never known about.

She learned.

When she told him that she was in the middle of a graduate program and that maybe she should become a nurse, he said, "Why don't you just finish what you started?"

This brilliant guy could finish a crossword puzzle in two minutes from a major newspaper and had never finished high school because on the first day in Frankford High, after Michael having gone to Catholic school, a student now stopped him in public school and told him he had to pay. And then Michael described how he punched the guy. And the discipline officer on that day said, "I guess I will be seeing a lot of you." But instead, Michael went to mechanical school and understood carpentry, plumbing, the boiler room, and electricity. He had a woman living with him, who, according to another woman, told her that she ran a beautiful house. She, who had not much, was in awe of his sensibilities, ideology, and witty kindness.

She had to light the candles for Hanukkah, a Jewish holiday with eight candles. She asked him to help and said, "You probably think this is ridiculous."

He said, "Listen, in the end, we all bleed and die."

She was on the roof looking at the star-studded sky, and he was climbing the water tower there. He said many people treated him differently. She thought she told him he was charismatic. He asked if that was what she was scared of. He leaned forward and was affectionate.

She said, "We're from different worlds," and he never let her ever forget that she had said that.

Michael would work three shifts straight and call her in the middle of the night to talk and tell her he wanted to be a football player, on that third shift, he would read the bible.

She got to go on a date with him in Frankford, a

working-class area of Philadelphia. The exotic feeling of this whole setting was fascinating. He then confessed at that bar that "The most important thing" in his life was "Jesus Christ."

When she used the word love to him at that biker's bar, which he called "Death Row," and while he was playing Bon Jovi on the jukebox, he explained the words, and his girlfriend had moved away before this happened.

She said the word love and how she had never used that word before. He had said, "Don't give me that word."

A rental agent got hired, and Michael got switched to the day shift. After that, she heard that she was chasing him around the building and telling him not to smoke.

Before that, her neighbor and best friend had gone out with the rental agent. The rental agent liked her own different combinations of drinks.

"She had fallen off the chair." The other had told that story after a new owner was hired, and the rental agent had lost a job.

Michael continued his friendship with her, which consisted of three times a week at fancy bars for two hundred dollars a day. . .She treated.

As the reader can imagine, this grated upon the woman and made her lovesick. His mother would tell the woman that he would go home and watch "How It's Made," which fascinated her because after fixing things, he went home to watch how things are made.

This was his passion. He was truly blessed. He would fix things for his neighbors' houses- pro bono.

He also understood the older women in the building; he just had that kind of emotional intelligence.

The week before the rental agent took him out

for his birthday, he told his mother about the woman, "Say hello to your future daughter-in-law."

The woman never missed a day of work but cried and talked to anyone who would listen after he had suddenly begun going out with the rental agent.

In all the talking that the woman did, she received two pieces of advice that were full of great wisdom:

Once, she received knowledge in a bar called "McClinchey's." A man told her that endings were always tragic. Looking back on that statement, the woman thought of Lady Colin Campbell's statement, "A lot of people don't want the discomfort of . . .independent thought and finding your unique way to light; they don't want to be spiritually or emotionally challenged or personally challenged, they want easy lives." The man in "McClinchey's" bar in Philadelphia was getting his Ph.D. in religion at Temple University.

Another piece of advice she received was from a garbage collector who told the woman, "You better get hold of yourself." Again, Lady Colin continued, stating, "Courageous people have learned to use fear." This man also had given her that advice in "McClinchey's."

One day at the job, a fellow mechanic told the woman that Michael was a good man who helped people of all cultures; he had no prejudice. She knew.

Each day, the woman would see them -her blond hair, his red hair at the lush bars around this lush place where the woman lived, and finally, the woman knew what the woman had to do.

One day, the woman walked over into the lush bar where they were sitting. Of course, the woman looked damn good. He walked over to her and asked the woman to join them. The woman made up her mind to show that she was upset with the rental agent and how much it grated upon the woman. That evening in the bar, the rental agent said, "I would ask you out too." In other words, she was trying to be nice.

Six months later, he called and told the woman, "It's over. Do you want this? I have a lot of problems."

And she said yes.

She continued working in teaching, which was difficult in regard to the unpredictable behaviors, which made one feel a rueful empathy for the policemen. The woman cared about the people and literary content, but it was the behaviors. As time passed, the woman was blessed with a pension.

On Thursdays and Sundays, his phone would go dead, and the woman would talk to his mother, who was a Born Again Christian and was putting in a prayer to the "700 Club" that the rental agent would leave town because his mother felt he was drinking more.

His mother was a calming oasis, a sense of normalcy amidst strife, and she really believed firmly. Michael had hooked up the phone so that the television would light up with the woman's or anyone's name when the woman called. The mother, who was a relief to talk with, would say that his mechanics had outsmarted the others. He said, "Well, yous both can talk," but the woman always pretended she never talked with the mother. One can see "13 Ways to Lose a Guy" to know why the woman knew not to tell him that she talked to the mother.

The mother used terms the woman hadn't heard except in her nineteenth-century novels from those small areas within the big city neighborhoods. For instance, "like that there." The woman told him she had outsmarted him with the mechanics of the television and his phone, and he said, "You ain't outsmarted no one."

Anthropologically, she had the best of both

worlds, the mother as spy and the son like a Damon Runyan character he was.

The mother said how he would run out the door at three years old to watch men fix cars and had learned it all. He would see someone fixing a roof, think they were doing it wrong, and join in. When he got hired at the high-rise, the owner told the maintenance head that he seemed "scrappy."

"Is he good?" The owner was told that Michael was good.

Then, the mother began to lose her memory.

According to the mother, Michael had decided to let the ex-rental agent move in to care for the mother. One must note the irony here- the mother had been praying to the "700 Club" that the rental agent would move away, and then the ex-rental agent moved into the mother's house. Well, sometimes God says no. Had the mother not told the woman, she would have never known.

The mother told the woman she should stop pining after him. The mother told the woman that the rental agent had just moved in, made hot dogs, and slept in another room. The rental agent did things three times after she would be drinking, the mother had said.

Here is the part of the story that the woman hopes he will not find from this story. His mother told the woman after she could not reach him for several days: "Guess who moved in?"

The ex-rental agent had moved in, the third time repeated, and the mother told the woman that there were vodka bottles all over the house.

One week later, the woman called the mother, and the sobbing mother told the woman that he had a stroke at 55. The mother and the ex-rental agent went to visit him daily. Then he was back to work, and he needed another operation.

By now, the mother had passed away, and the ex-rental agent lived with him. The woman asked whether the rental agent drank, and he said she did every few days and that he himself was planning to drink some beers…

There were seven feral cats in the back of the house, and the ex-rental agent was feeding them, the mother had said.

The woman was then in isolation due to the pandemic- away from the building where she lived in Philadelphia. She spoke with him on the nights when he came to work, but the phone was dead when he was at home. Maybe she'll stay in the little town. "I'm not no side jaune," the students would say.

And so, it went. She was resolved to read James Joyce's "Ulysses," with explanatory volumes, after being at her mother's house with her deceased father's book collection, who was an English professor until he was 91 when he retired as pictured.

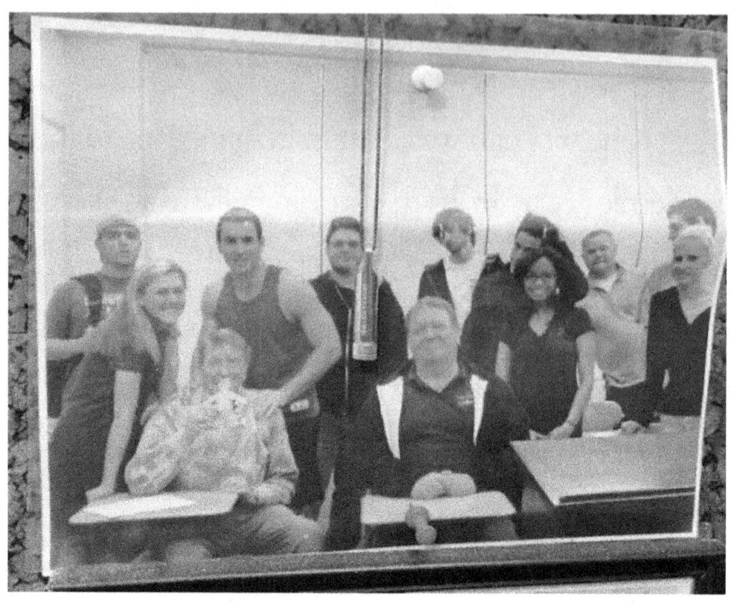

This is what her father Monro, in the above
picture with a class when he was 91 years old, with
the tan shirt and sitting in the front, said: one must
read the explanatory books with ancient text or
convoluted text, and that includes graphic novels and
Cliff Notes on the text.

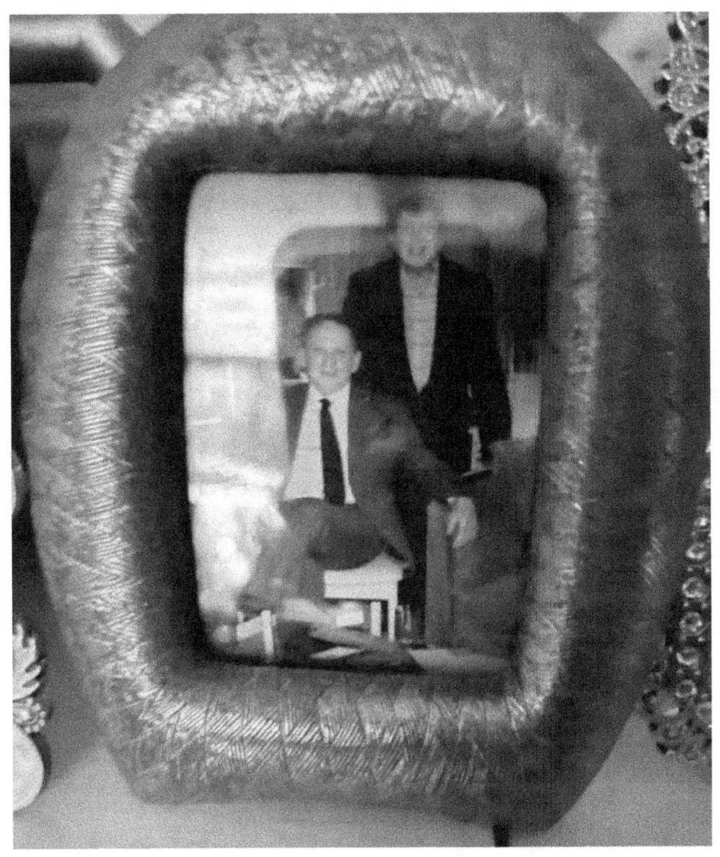

So, with complex texts or novels, the allusion was that Aristotle said that life depends on setting and time, and removing the scenery did help the situation.

In the woman's life was Uncle Harold, who was a clever guy who liked gambling and patterned himself after his maternal cousin once removed,

Philip Gunczenberger.

Harold's girlfriend, when his wife had left, Sandy, when the woman had approached her during the pandemic at a restaurant bar, Sandy said, "Oh, you are a liberal," in response to the woman wearing a mask.

Sandy would be at the opulent bar where Mimi, her friend Shirley, and the woman would go each week. Sandy would bend her elbow and drink martinis with her friend, Rita, who owned "The Shanty," named after the expression that there are two types of Irish shanty and lace curtain.

Sandy had spoon-fed Helen Roth during Helen's last illness when no family member could. She said later, "I don't do funerals," to the request of Mimi to come to Monro's funeral. Mimi was miffed, and she would say hello and walk through. The woman would remember the parties with Harold and Sandy. On the mantel had been a picture of

Teddy Kennedy, and Harold would say to Sandy, "He and his wife are just like us; she drinks, he cheats." And Sandy would be steaming. Monro wrote the speech for Sandy's parents' 50th anniversary at the Italian club downtown, among others, and then the mayor of Allentown asked to buy the speech.

Sandy leaned forward one night to the woman and said, "Listen, don't tell your mother, but having grandchildren is the best."

In pandemic times, Sandy's loyalties had changed to a more conservative bent with Trump as president, and as she bent her elbow, she talked politics in a firecracker way.

She was a pistol, a real entertainment for Harold. Her son had met a Korean woman who was built like a brick-bit house, and he was in love.

Harold was giving him advice about his thriving appliance store, and as the Korean woman could finally speak English, he fell out of love just like in the "South Pacific" movie's song, "Happy Talk."

Mimi's friend Shirley loved her boots and jewelry and gave parties at a chemical company. She was a real lady, but she, too, refused the vaccine. She did beat the illness but not the son, but there became a wound from her boots, one of her great passions. That is the horror when passions do one in. Sandy and her son Joey did not get the vaccine. Sadly, Sandy passed at a young age several months later with her son an owner of an appliance store. Both had not taken the vaccine.

Harold's other niece did not respond one night at the restaurant when he had asked her where she was going next, so he responded, "I just want to know where not to go." When the woman informed him that her father Monro had told her that she should move to the smaller town of Northampton for school, he said, "No, it wouldn't help."

Her father, who had a sudden illness at 92 after working until 91, had told her about Thomas Wolfe's poem "Do Not Go Gentle." Rather than the "gently" adverb, the "gentle" is an adjective and a clue for interpretation. The adjective "gentle" modifies the understood "you." "Gentle you, do not go," is the interpretation. Thomas Wolfe had said, "You got a 50% chance of getting to an Afterlife, you might as well believe," is what Monro explained in his last six weeks of life. Harold, who acted like the "bad boy" but had a kind heart, explained once at a party that he was surprised he had lived so long until 87 years of age. He had worked for hours with his father, Abe, at the Roth Brothers' furniture store. Once, Helen, the mother, said that Harold had a broken leg that years later Harold had never known about.

Monro said he did believe. Once, he asked when her sibling was ill, "Do you pray?" and she asked, "Do you believe?" He, too, had said yes. Really, what he also had said then in 1974 was that he didn't understand why, when there were people hooked up by tubes in hospitals, other people would want to take illegal drugs. This is what he said to the woman as she resolved not to do that.

The woman went to the Czech Republic and then to Slovakia to meet Alex Roth, Jr., and viewed his determination, not wanting to view the prayer paper; but then he took a picture of the prayer after she had prayed in front of Alex's grandfather's grave. Alex Jr., had gone through the Soviets' occupying the Czech Republic and having his religion and relatives both decimated, and now he watched the video of himself that the woman had created of him.

In the story "Memory Fields: The Legacy of a Wartime Childhood in Czechoslovakia," Author Shlomo Breznitz, who hid in a Catholic Seminary in Bratislava, near Vysna Jablonka, Writer and Psychologist Breznitz, said that boys would come up to him and say, "Let me see your eyes."

Author Breznitz, who would become a psychologist, would answer back, "Let me see your eyes. Are you Jewish?"

He survived and went to visit the nun who had hidden him. John Josco, a relative of Zuzana, within Jan Augusta's booklets about her family in Vysna Jablonka, John Josco would describe how, after being orphaned, he and his brothers lived in an orphanage and ran away to a farmhouse. In 1899, they came to get him with horses and carriages...

Alex Jr. looked so seriously at himself on the video, and she asked, "Do you think you look good?"

Kata, Jr. translated, and he nodded, "Yes." He said that he thought he looked good. Thoughtfully, he said that he had to get an I-13 phone. Ursula, his German descent wife, so beautiful and helpful, had her genealogy notebooks ready for all the relatives in Humenne.

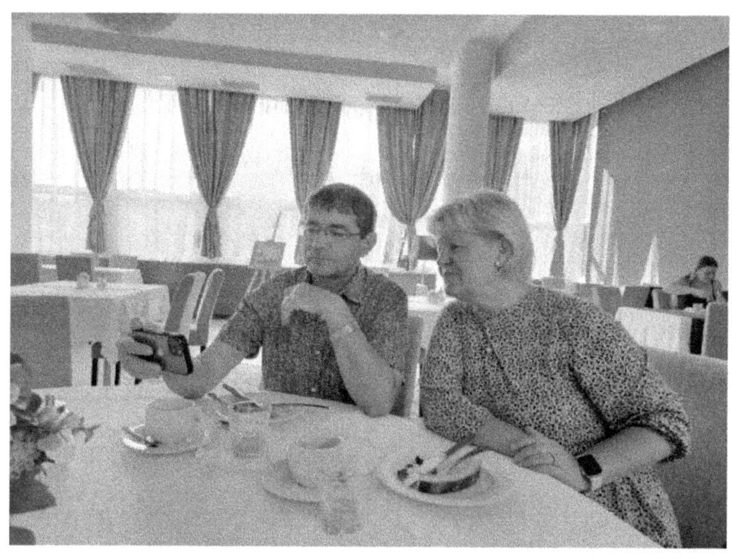

The woman recalled when her father Monro would look in the mirror and say, "Boy, am I a good-looking guy!" There was a stark reminder between Alex the woman's newly discovered second cousin, and Monro, the woman's father.

Alex, Jr. and Ursula met through Ursula's relative, and the relative had arranged for Alex, Jr. to do engineering work in her house. The relatives were setting up that Alex would be there when Ursula would be at the apartment. Suddenly, there was music; Alex and Ursula began to dance, and when the music stopped, they kept dancing, Kata Jr. said.

They said this after the woman asked how they had met.

Similarities of the character traits of what would have been Monro's first cousin once removed were uncanny. Monro took the "e" off his name, had it legally changed, and placed this information in the newspaper, much to the banter of others.

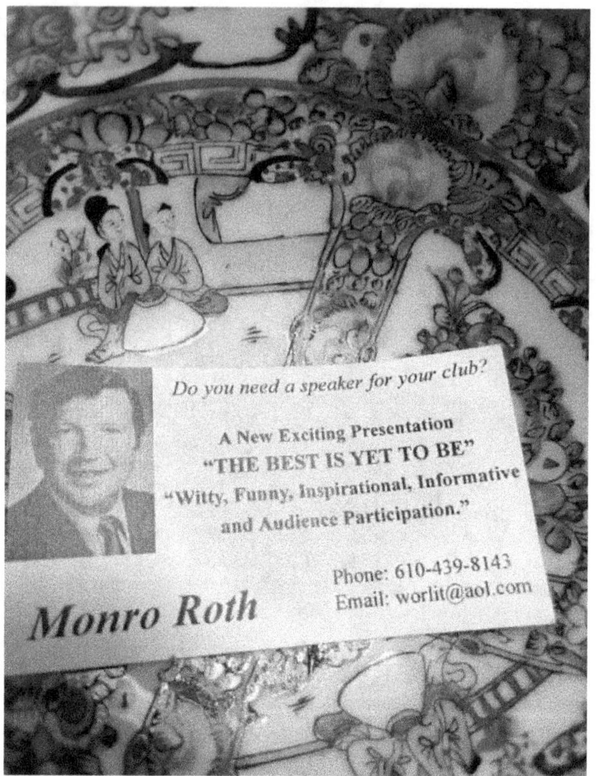

God, Kindness, and Switching the Setting
through a World's Catastrophe are antidotes for
people here.

The woman liked people who had varied
perspectives on life and had a Platonic male
colleague. He chose to live in a difficult
neighborhood. He rode his bike to work, ate rice and

vegetables, never missed a Mass, and would walk over stones to help someone in need or who was troubled.

He counseled and got counseling for his various family members who were scarily out of control with addiction while he was never missing a day of work.

But he often had these "would-have, could-have, should-have" dilemmas about career, purpose of life, romance, and human alliances. Like many other humans, he had one other fatal flaw. He would question the woman, "What if I marry and then meet a better person after I marry her?"

This was an interesting dilemma, so the woman queried many people about this. The woman began with her father, Monro, and her mother, Mimi. Both said in their ways that they just hit it off with each other, and they just knew.

The woman then enquired to a best friend and psychologist, Carol, who had recently married, and she responded that "there is always that risk, and if that happens, that happens, but in the meanwhile, she and her husband trust each other since they have talked."

Well, fast forward to when the woman's Platonic male friend had trouble at work, an unfair evaluation. Well, the woman he was dating at the time offered him to go into business with her salon.

So, the other woman said to him, "Listen, you can always look at women; you can even flirt, but my mother, Mimi, says that it is 'better to face the world with two than one.'"

Then the woman told him this: "She," his girlfriend, "faced something with you at your most forlorn moment in life, so why don't you just try?"

The woman also believed that she had added that he did not have to tell her everything about what he was thinking or even doing. The woman believed she was thinking of "Bridges of Madison County" when the woman said that because in that movie, not the book, the character met someone after marriage.

Well, the woman's friend made the decision and married her. At that time, he kept two separate residences within their neighborhood. The woman, feeling that she had accommodated his preference, shared with him the story of Simone De Beauvoir in "The Second Sex" and her existentialist companion, Sartre, about how they both had chosen to live eight blocks apart.

At the wedding of her friend whom she had given advice to, the wife's family appeared in exquisite silk robes, representing their Asian heritage. They took this occasion seriously, as the woman was informed, while the husband's relatives hailed from England, including his English aunt, who had married an aristocrat. The woman engaged her in a conversation about Jane Austen within the nave of the North Philadelphian Catholic church.

Lately, the woman noticed a newfound maturity in her Platonic friend. He genuinely seemed to care about his new wife. Wondering, she asked him if he were still inclined to explore relationships with other women or if he harbored concerns about finding someone better.

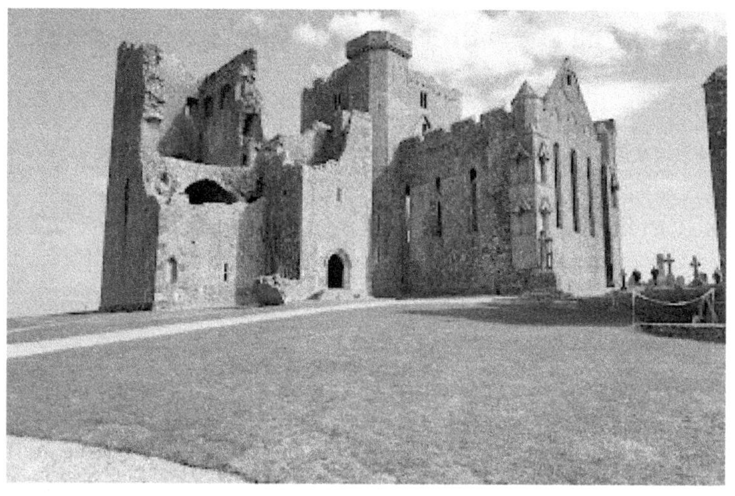

To her surprise, he responded,

"That would not be fair to her."

The woman was astonished by this change of heart and perspective, especially since she considered that her own advice was not exactly rooted in personal experience but rather in secondhand information.

The irony lay in the fact that he had aged like a fine wine, infused with a touch of wisdom as well.

This had been a colleague, yet the workplace and the social place together was what the woman usually avoided, especially the workplace party, unless it were politically expedient.

Amid the woman's work, though, once, at the jewelry company, Mario remarked, "You've got pathos, drama, and humor, so don't mock it." This comment was prompted by the woman's surprise when she witnessed individuals laughing at a magazine picture.

On another occasion, a student commented, "But we argue with all of our teachers this way."

The woman found herself attending a teacher's party at the Electrical Union's building on Second and Mifflin Streets in South Philadelphia. Despite her usual reluctance to socialize with colleagues, she had been employed at a vocational school for twelve years, and she did have one exception.

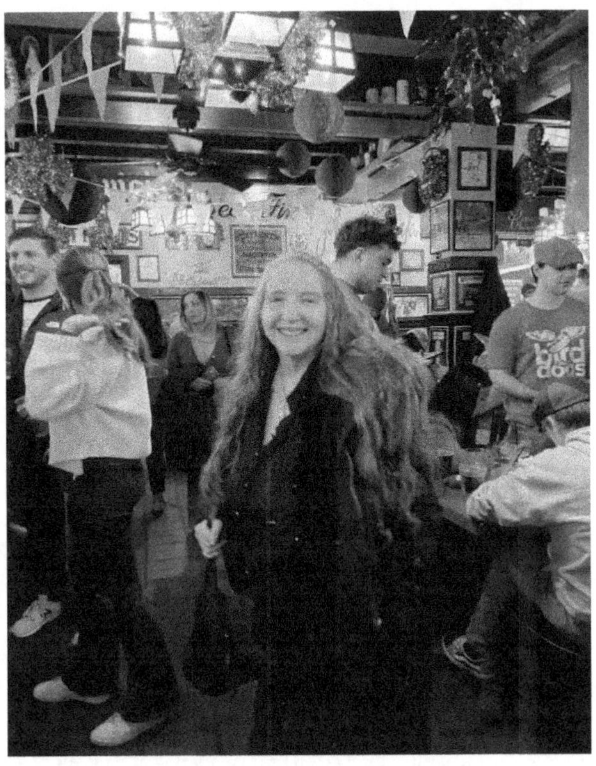

She would only go with colleagues to a party if it were a good business policy to do so.

Marguerite Duras once said, "No other human beings, no woman, no poem or music, book or painting can replace alcohol in its power to give man the illusion of real creation."

Well, creation and illusion were happening

amidst employees here. Among the teachers at her school. There was one who stood out in her eyes; he was not only a teacher but a carpenter as well. The combination added to his appeal, making him the only person throughout her years of teaching who truly captivated her. Her best friend once mentioned a quote from Marguerite Duras, "Alcohol leads to unknown passages."

Well, despite her wariness, some insisted that she try an apple martini. She ended up having many, which made her inebriated afterward. The imagery of the scene is not something any person needs to be privy to. She ended up being ill near bathroom walls after he drove her home. No romantic involvement had occurred, nor would have, but she found herself scrubbing walls the following evening.

Donning a black leather jacket and cowboy boots, he had a striking appearance. She, too, possessed a charm of her own, although she usually made an effort not to be noticed at school.

The next day, the secretary at the school, a true South Philly local who dabbled in witchery and had even performed belly dancing in Egypt, received a call informing her that the handsome teacher would not be coming to work.

Curiosity piqued, the secretary asked, "What did you do to him?"

Everyone had observed her leaving with him, in a direction opposite to the "Walk of Shame," as he offered her a ride. She replied, "We did nothing," to which the secretary playfully retorted, "I would have."

If one is paying close attention, dear reader, this is a tale of her Female Guile, akin to a jar of nuts in a coffee shop.

She not only refrained from getting romantically involved with colleagues but also took time with a courtship while keeping her romance separate from the workplace.

The woman's parents, Monro and Mimi, said they had met through a jeweler, Paul Lobel, and saw each other at "Chock Full of Nuts" in New York when he went to college after World War II. On weekends, he worked for his father Abe's store in Northampton, Pennsylvania.

While in his 90s, Monro's two stories to his classes were of him dipping the girls' curls in the inkwell and of the time when he walked over to the wall and started drawing on the walls. His high school, Northampton High, was a small-town place where immigrants' children in 1941 thrived and had bands-he played solo clarinet and saxophone, and he and his sister had won an oratory prize. His cousin Joel Roth and sibling Shirley Roth wrote a play.

Before going to World War II, Monro was stationed in Ohio, where his mother Helen came by train and brought a military-style coat. As Monro later rode the train with the jacket on, he noticed people were saluting to him. Before this, in the Rialto theatre in Allentown on D Day, the lights came on, and it was announced in 1941 that America was at war, and Helen began to sob because Monro would serve. Meanwhile Joel and Shirley would sit by the river and read the classics out loud to each other.

In World War II, Monro won an award for bravery, and when telling an interviewer for a newspaper about meeting his wife, he spoke of her coming to the Poconos' arena with a midriff on and then said, "Enough said." Who knew? Too much Philip Roth's writings, maybe. He was an expert in that writing and taught about him until he was 91.

Meanwhile, Mimi, the daughter of a psychiatrist who would become violent and who had a patient- daughter of Marlene Dietrich who was trying to change her affinity for the same sex- with Mimi's father as her psychiatrist, well Mimi was busy liking this Monro.

In the 1950s, Mimi had traveled to Cuba with three "gals," as she called them, and recalled the huge statue of Fidel Castro.

Now, in 1953, Mimi would wait for Monro to pass the coffee shop "Chock Full of Nuts" in New York, and he would wave and walk on. The woman surmised Mimi was seeking things she could not have back then.

She had wanted to be an actress, so she went to Summer Stock in Newport, Rhode Island, and gave Zachery Scott, an actor, an intestinal problem after she had served him a drink on stage.

Mimi and Zelda would follow Helen Hayes

from the Broadway shows to Ms. Hayes' place. Her mother, Zelda, came to Mimi's Summer Stock camp and said, "You want to act?" This was after Mimi was assigned to scrubbing toilets, "Do it on your own time." In a camp before this, Zelda, who was busy working in Russicks' store, fabricated what happened with a radio show, "Elsa Clench," and told Mimi the made-up version after she had gone to childhood camp.

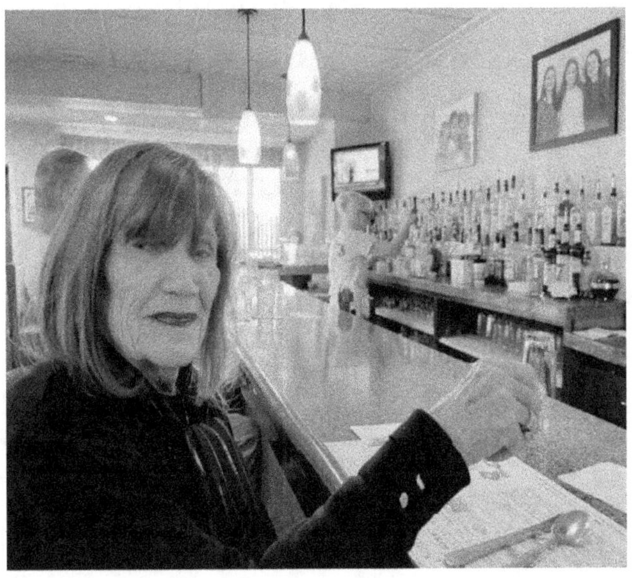

This is when Mimi is 94, after her daughter convinces her to sit at the bar of a local restaurant,

"Werts." The woman used to assure Zelda and Bea that Mimi got to apply her acting in her daily life, or as her father Monro once said, "Every woman is a Machiavellian." Or as was stated in the film, "Two Can Play the Game," one male character said, "The F.B.I. and the C.I.A. don't have anything over a woman with a plan." During Mimi's wedding, Sam Rubin, founder of "Faberge Perfumes," played piano in Zelda's apartment, where Monro's two first cousins once removed, Berta and Edith Nieman, both daughters of Anna Chaimovsova Niemanova who were Chaimovics came. But cousins were supposed to not be invited, but Monro thought they were "aunts," and that caused a brouhaha with Shapiro cousins on Mimi's side who were not invited.

Later, she met Monro at Tamiment, a Wilkes Barre country entertainment area, again and gave him an ultimatum. . .

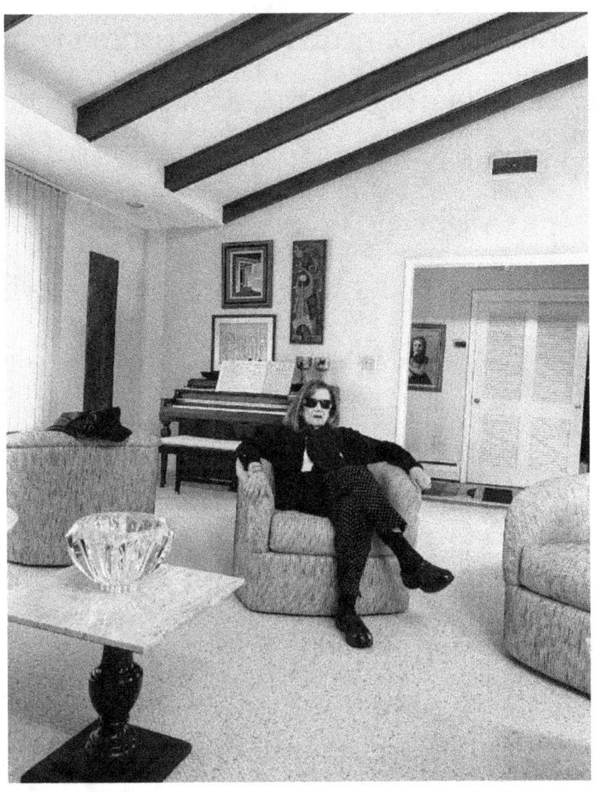

She got her way.

The carpentry teacher told the woman later that he realized she was "shy" and was different from what he had thought.

She would never forget the party. She never missed a day in 30 years of teaching.

Another one of her rules during meetings was to never raise one's hand. Instead, she took a different approach when she was sharing the "shittah," referring to light and trivial matters, as opposed to "dichta," which encompassed the deeper and more profound topics.

However, there was rarely any time for discussions in inner-city schools. The staff and maybe even the students were in a state of siege, reminiscent of the last three years of middle school in the city's northern parts. In Frankford, right next to Michael's house, incidents such as a BB gun being discovered on a young female student happened. North of the Center City, a flickering fire of a lighter on the floor while the woman emphatically slammed a Tennessee Williams' book on it, or in Frankford, an emotionally distressed student pushing desks down during an actual lockdown, was the atmosphere of constant turmoil.

Now, she found herself at a party, where she

spontaneously climbed onto a chair after Ron, a department head, encouraged this, and she began to dance. At that moment, she had no awareness of where her purse was, nor was she concerned about that. The carpentry teacher, being chivalrous, said, "Sit here. I'm a corner man." She couldn't help but find his gesture cool and charming.

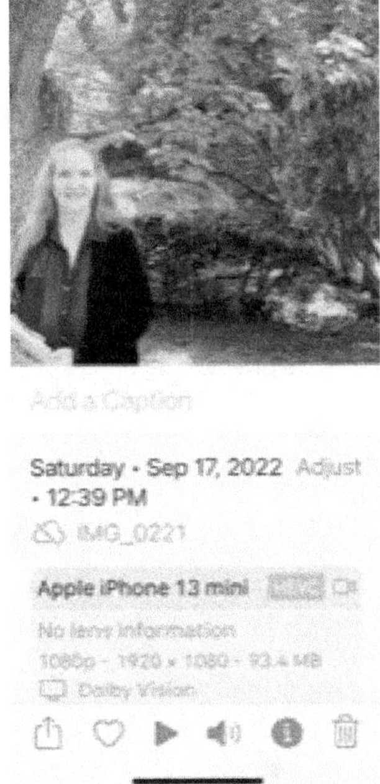

Soon after, she needed a gentle departure from work, which a friend considered as "nothing more than a mere inconvenience." In fact, she now held

two jobs, and so she was working seven days a week.
Unexpectedly, her Aunt Lucille sent her a sum of
two thousand dollars, accompanied by a request not
to visit Atlantic City.

Up until that point, Atlantic City had served as
her escape, where she would stroll the boardwalk and
spend fifty dollars on a quarter poker machine. Every
now and then, she would win, and the winnings
would pay her student loan.

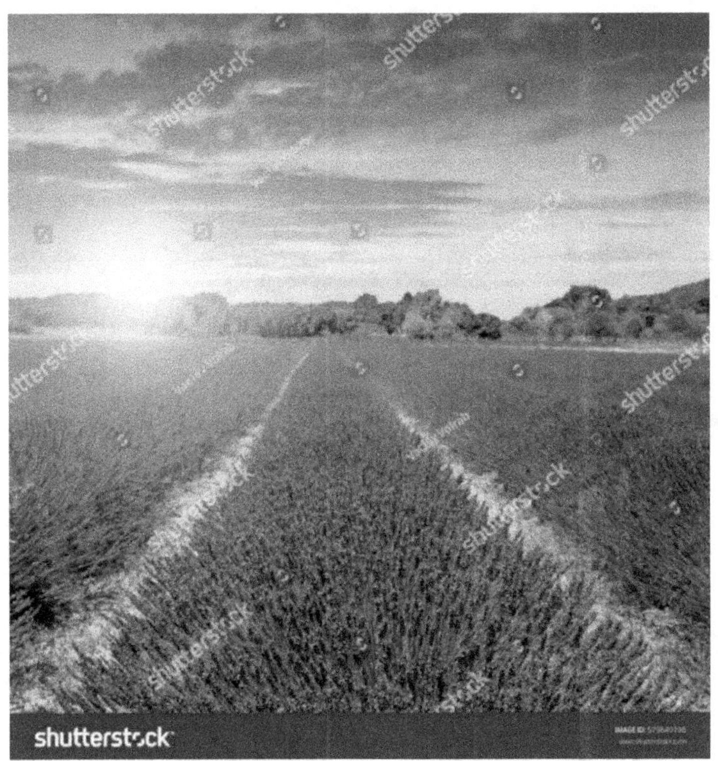

She embarked on a trip to Ireland with the two thousand dollars she received. Her parents introduced her to a credit card and the guided tour.

Later, her tour guide displayed knowledge of Ireland. He shared bits with tourists, such as the presence of Hawthorne trees growing in the middle of fields amidst farmland. Farmers refused to cut down these trees because they served as burial sites for babies from the famine of 1848.

1848 was a year for a census being taken of every family amidst the Hapsburg Empire in Europe. And now, this famine in Ireland was described carefully.

Another story he told involved a mechanic refusing to remove a church's cross on an outer wall that was being repurposed for a new hotel. Will Collins, the tour guide, taught the tourists not to say "goodbye" but rather, "Till we meet again."

The guide informed the tourists that according to local folklore, a girl who spotted three white horses would supposedly find herself getting married. The woman knew she was in the land of Lillian Hellman's perspective where in "Pentimento,"…

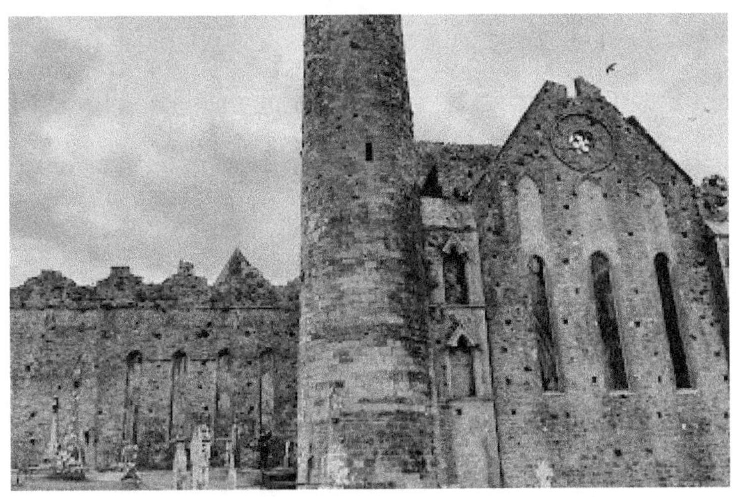

...the writer finds "spirituality in all places." With the guide who worked in anthropology at Limerick University, the tourists were taken to the outer edge of Limerick, where the "Traveling People" had acquired wealth by collecting discarded wooden furniture from hotels. However, their illiteracy led to their "To Let" signs hanging upside down.

This anthropology professor further explained that the "Traveling People" understood how to cure an eye infection of an animal when the veterinarians could not. The woman had learned about "Travelers," formerly "Gypsies," through finely written stories in Irish newspapers that she read during her visits to taverns in small villages. There, in one small town of Sligo, the tourists on a bus saw a "Travelers'" funeral caused by a love rivalry between two sects of "Traveling People."

During the Irish tour, at nighttime, the woman found herself at a castle where medieval enactments were taking place. Mead was a corn liquor in literature found in "Beowulf," an Old English epic poem from 700 A.D. She had mead, which was being served during the night excursions in Ireland. The "epic" nature of the poem was created by formal language of alliteration, superheroes, and conflicts and could explain characters in the castle performing and acting out these medieval writings within the night excursions in Ireland.

She also recalled liquor's mention in "The Canterbury Tales," a literary work from 1387 A.D., written in Middle English and often read with a German-like accent. In that tale, characters embark on a pilgrimage to a shrine. In the 1300's, the English were still Catholic before Henry the VIII in the late 1500's had changed the sect.

However, on this night in 2005 A.D., the woman became tipsy with mead, leading to a different kind of mentality.

The change made her vow to no longer drink hard liquor.

The following day, the tour guide continued to share how Irish people value the sacredness of the land arrangement and how the government prohibits malls in the Republic of Ireland. He explained how farmers received pensions and new homes from the European Union.

She was so mystically enchanted that she did not want to return to America nor leave the tour nor the guides.

But then, at the Irish airport, she felt a sense of an otherworldly moment as she realized the need for towns to balance farming, woodlands, and human settlements to preserve fauna and forestry.

Just then, an airport employee approached her with an offer to stay an extra day, which would give her a hotel, meals, and $500, all in the year 2005, during her financially challenging times.

Amazed, she accepted and spent the day interviewing redheads and writing their stories with photographs.

Upon her return to Philadelphia, she visited the casino by bus, played poker slots, and still in Irish wonder won $1000. She gave $500 for gifts and used the remaining $1000 to pay her student loan.

Despite being back in Philadelphia, she had now begun her loyalty to Ireland and would return each summer for tours, where she would sing and bring along Irish music.

After a woman praised this by saying, "You live life with purpose." following a performance, she spoke with a music teacher on the bus from Nova Scotia, who responded, "reasonably." Living a purposeful life seemed right.

Throughout her experiences, she learned lessons: Firstly, refraining from going out for drinks with colleagues was best, although attending parties for political reasons was necessary. Secondly, discussing romantic alliances should be avoided in work settings. Lastly, swearing off drinking hard liquor was a happening for her.

However, as one era in her life drew to a close and retirement from the workforce became a possibility, she discovered the freedom to pursue her passions. Genealogy became one of her interests, leading her to take the Ancestry D.N.A. test. The first close match she found was on her mother's side; that match revealed a second cousin from her maternal grandmother's lineage.

For the woman's mother, a first cousin once removed appeared on Mimi's Shapiro side. Shapiro translated to spear maker from Spain's Golden Age. Mimi's mother, Zelda, had siblings named Morris, Rose, and Bea. Statistics revealed a 40% mortality rate among other lost siblings in the early twentieth century, with causes of death including pneumonia, appendicitis, and rheumatic fever. Morris had married Rose who held the position of president of the New York School District. Rose even appeared on "The Virginia Graham Show" and worked for Governor Rockefeller, maybe because of her brother's influence, who owned Faberge.

Mimi and her lifelong best friend Scotty who is 95 years old as of 2024, were told by their teacher that they would land up in jail. This was told to them in second grade when they had gotten into a fistfight because Mimi had touched Scotty's pasted-down hair clip; Mimi claimed she wanted to see if the hair would move back. Then, Mimi went by the name Mignon, and Scotty, Hortense, which later transformed into Scotty, and Mignon into Mimi due to classmates pronouncing the "g." Another exploit was that Scotty would leave class and place a cigarette in the telephone pole, and Mimi would follow her there.

Scotty's mother lived to be over a hundred years old, and one pastime was strolling the streets of New York City in a thread-bare dress. On one occasion, Scotty's mother struck up a conversation with a cafeteria customer, boasting about his fashion designer son, Ralph Lauren. But at the moment of discussion, Scotty's mother refused to move her chair to sit with Ralph Lipshitz.

Recently, Scotty, on a visit to Mimi's house, revealed a clue in genealogy. She told the story of an uncle who had changed his age on the ship to America, and she also revealed how they had gone to California and had to share one bed with both working different work shifts. Could this be similar to the situations in Kolbasov and Vysna Jablonka in the early twentieth century?

The man near Scotty's mother's seat in the New York café expressed frustration because his son had changed his last name to Lauren.

Meanwhile, Zelda had promised Mimi that she would listen to the radio soap opera with Elsa Clench while Mimi went to overnight camp. However, Zelda was occupied with a sales job at Russicks, so she would make up stories about the events in Elsa Clench's radio show.

In 1974, Rose approached Scotty in Mimi's den. Scotty's mother had little money, but Scotty's husband had established a seasoning sauce factory, and they now owned horses.

Rose, curious about Scotty's life, asked, "What do you do?" To which Scotty, with a twinkle in her eyes and dimples sparkling, replied, "Anything I want." Rose was piqued.

Rose's brother had founded Faberge, and his companion was involved with the production of "No, No Nanette."

Fifty years later, still vibrant and twinkling-eyed, Scotty now has a 100-year-old gentleman friend. In contrast, one of her daughters chooses not to have a boyfriend at her daughter's request, while the other daughter declares she would never remarry if her current marriage were to end. As of now, Scotty's red-haired grandchildren have not yet had children.

Rose's brother had founded Faberge. Morris and Rose had a son and a daughter who went to Middlebury College. Jimmy was in "The Bohemian Club" in the 1950's. Within five months, he made two women pregnant.

The woman met in 2019 the newly discovered two children of Jimmy, the granddaughter and grandson of Rose and Morris. But all of their lives, the relatives knew nothing about these two children.

Jimmy's daughter informed the woman about a distressing incident that occurred at Morris' and Rose's doorstep. At the time, Rose was involved with an organization that was supposed to help discourage young people from taking drugs. Rose used to be picked up by a limousine to do that job. The incident at the doorstep involved a woman who had been promised a ring and marriage. It's worth noting that the children involved in this situation have now grown up.

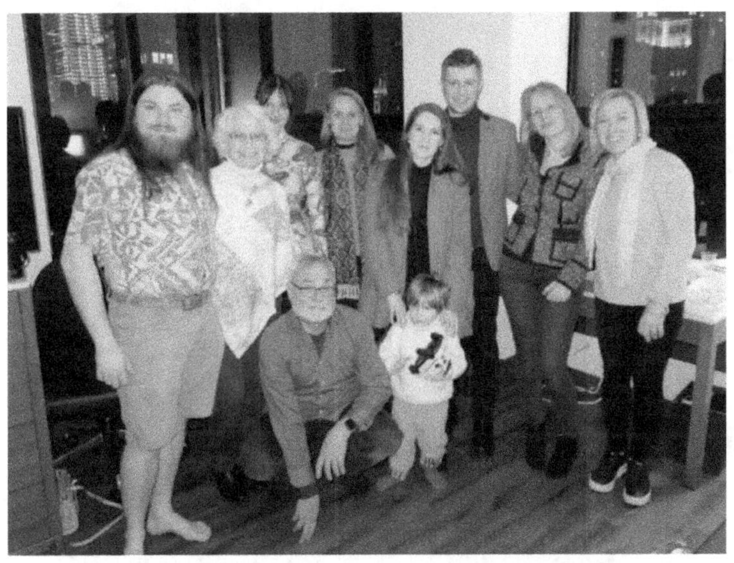

The woman has now become friends with the two children from Jimmy's two liaisons, and the children from the two liaisons are friends with the children of the late wife. The woman believes Darwin's "Survival of the Fittest Has No Morality." Rather not that there is no morality, as Darwin said, but that she thinks that siblings can have a harmonious relationship even if their mothers be rivals.

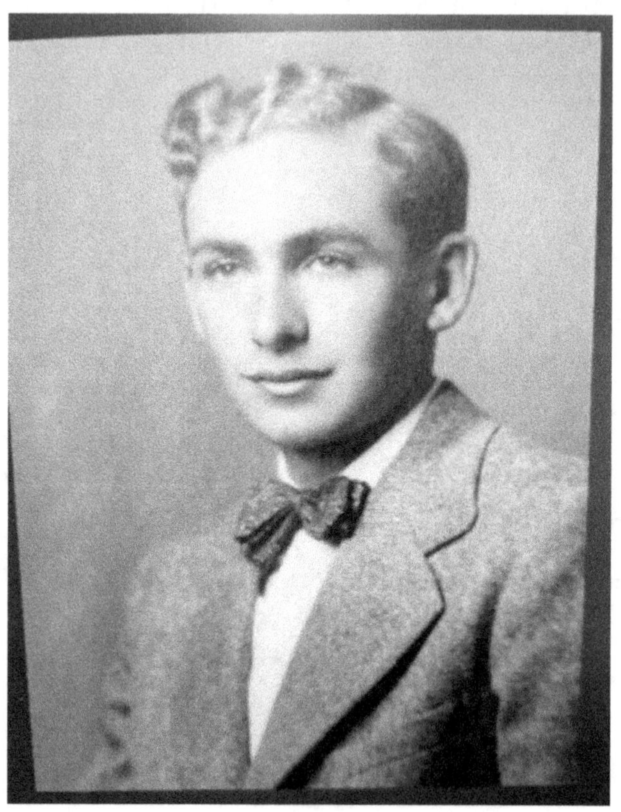

Jimmy, as in the picture above, was an apparent catnip for some women. His wife met the two other children after he had passed, and then she, Pia, who was Swedish and made those big heaping breaths of air for "yes," turned his ashes behind the books on the bookshelf.

He was a pilot in the Navy. He supposedly worked for the C.I.A., and his daughter, from a liaison, coincidentally worked for the N.S.A.

On the father's side, Monro's mother's mother and Mimi's father's father are related. Mimi's father, Gottlieb, is described as causing Mimi to be 5th to 8th cousins with Monro due to his mother's mother, specifically on the Gunczenberger side. This close familial relationship could result in endogamy, which might lead to difficulties, yet there was no loss due to war or Shoah on the mother's side.

Marrying outside of tribes or religions might increase variability, which will increase the strength of the species, Charles Darwin, a biologist, said.

But as one laboratory coworker said, "There will be those few who cling to the bible."

The woman was already visiting the people of the villages of Vysna Jablonka and Kolbasov, and the woman had visited with the relatives discovered in 2019; then she visited in 2022. Isador had come to America in 1907, Abe, who came to America in 1910, and Joe, who came in 1925, all would go to the port and give money to their parents, Bernard Roth and his wife, Rosalie Chaimovicsova, Adele Roth Wolensky had said.

Bernard Roth had Isador, Abe, and Joe, who had all emigrated from Slovakia to Allentown, Pennsylvania.

In 1936, Joe went back courageously to tell his family to leave. He took a picture with people who have now been identified.

The one sister had six, but nine by 1942, children, who lived in Humenne in 1930 with Joe's father and mother. All refused to leave. The one brother of Joe, Jakub, had died a natural death of typhoid after working for a tavern in Solinka, Poland, in 1915. He has a grave in Humenne; he had a son who stayed and another son, Samuel Elias Roth, who survived.

That was the miracle. Though Tova Friedman, in her book, "Child of Auschwitz," who is Lucille Roth Lehrich's daughter's mother-in-law, states that Tova had said she survived through "luck," not "miracles," because the others had not "survived."

Zuzana's manager contacted the woman in 2019; the woman figured out that Zuzana's Jewish grandfather was Izrael Chaimovics, a first cousin to the woman's great-grandmother.

Jana states that Zuzana "went to school through the forests on foot from Vysna Jablonka to the town Snina 18.5 kilometers away. On Sunday," Zuzana "went to Snina, and on Friday, she returned home." She did not have shoes. This is similar to Helen Roth's brother, Max Roth, who said he walked three miles, according to his granddaughter Lynn, to school from Kolbasov and did not want to wear down his leather, so he walked with bare feet.

Jakub, the son of Bernard, who passed in 1915, had had a ticket, and that ticket had helped a family member from Helen's side to emigrate. Vlad, the son-in-law of Alex Jr., has just learned that both sides of Abe and Helen, who married in Allentown, both sides - Abe's side, who lived in Vysna Jablonka, and Helen's side, who lived in Kolbasov, knew each other after Abe and Helen had gotten married in Allentown in 1923.

The woman's father, Monro Roth, has a fascinating and mysterious family background. His mother, Helen, was originally named Roth, but the family changed it before the year 1869 from Moskovits to Roth in order to avoid conscription. There is a sense of intrigue, mystery, and exoticism surrounding Helen. The woman has made significant efforts to uncover the hidden secrets that emerged from this enigmatic family history.

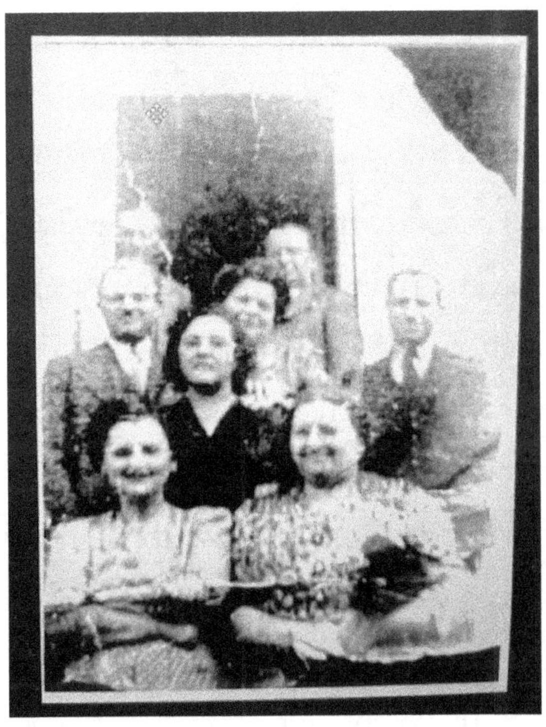

The woman in the black is Helen Roth in 1946.
Isador had now married the love of his life, Rose
Pachter, third row from the bottom. Helen is in the
second row. Her husband, Abe, is in the last row on
the right side from the viewer's view. Helen is near
Isador, who is right behind Helen in the third row
from the bottom, first on the left, viewer's point of

view.

In one of the stories of immigrants, there was a woman who, in 1924, was so isolated from not knowing the language that another man might have helped her get to the bigger city. Years later, the daughter of a child would take the test, and she would be from that father. That father was interested in poetry and music, and his son would write, and his daughter would play music, but the woman would be a favorite to the household father. There was a woman whose husband gambled, did not worry about his co-workers, and bought life insurance policies on his parents. He primped each day, dolled up in three-piece suits, and was seen with women other than his wife.

In 1924, a plate came out about Colonel Lindbergh, who later would fly to visit the leader Adolph Hitler, but meanwhile, in America he was a folk hero. There was a man who stayed with his parents and then revisited his parents and was

devastated by those life policies, and he had taken
sick.

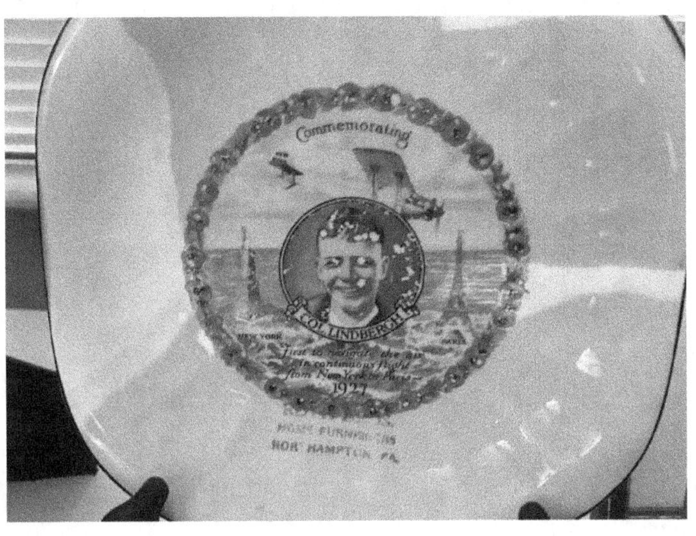

In 1936, four things happened: 1) the king of
England abdicated for the sake of love, 2) Lillie Weiss
died after giving Isador seven children, 3) Helen's
father died and got a grave in Kolbasov, and 4) Joe
went back to Vysna Jablonka to try to get his parents
out, his sister and what would be nine children by
1942, and his brother's two sons, and they all stayed.
They all refused to leave. They had a maid in
Michaelovce at that time that was listed in the 1930
Census as living with them.

In 1921, while on her ship, Helen was 20 years old, according to the civil document. However, she also mentioned that her first child, Monro, was born in 1923 when she said she was 16. The woman firmly believed in this account. But now there has been a document discovered of a civil record that proves that she was 20.

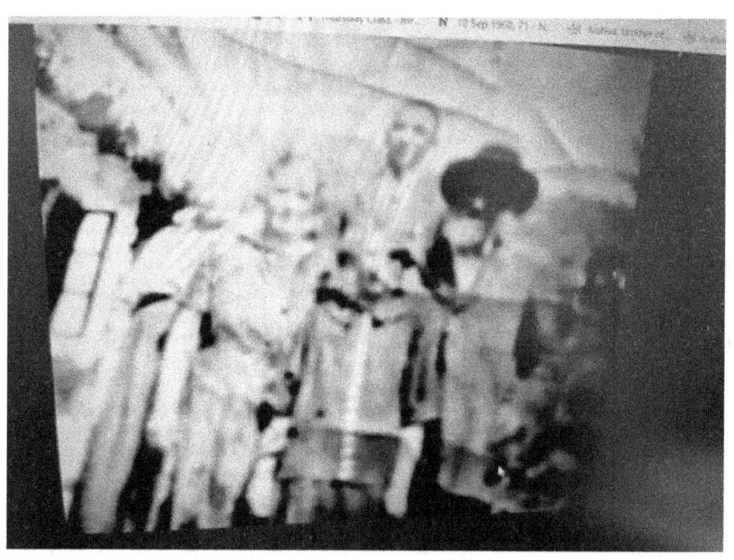

On the left side, from the viewer's point of view, on the above page is the older woman, slightly in the back, Rifka Gunczenberger Rothova from Sztarina. She is the only person not accounted with, in terms of her demise. the exception of what her granddaughter Shirley had said that Helen had said in regard to Rifka of an uncertain danger .

From the viewers' point of view, on the left is Lenka Roth in the bottom row, who was born in 1913. Then, in the most frontal point is Helena, born in 1915. Salamon Roth, a tall, slim guy in the back, was born in 1909. The older man with the white beard and black fedora was Samuel Moses Roth, born in 1864. His father, Wolf Moskovits, had his name changed from Moskovits to Roth to avoid conscription.

Samuel Moses Roth born in 1864 in the 1930 Census lists his birth place as Zboj. In the 1869 Czechoslovakian Census in Zboj provided by JewishGen.Org, there is a Farkus Roth, with a child named Mosko Roth born in 1864 in Zboj, the same year of birth as Samuel Moses Roth's birth. Samuel Moses Roth's father was a Wolf Moskovits who changed his name from Moskovits to Roth,

according to relatives Shirley, Carol, Lynn, and
Lucille.

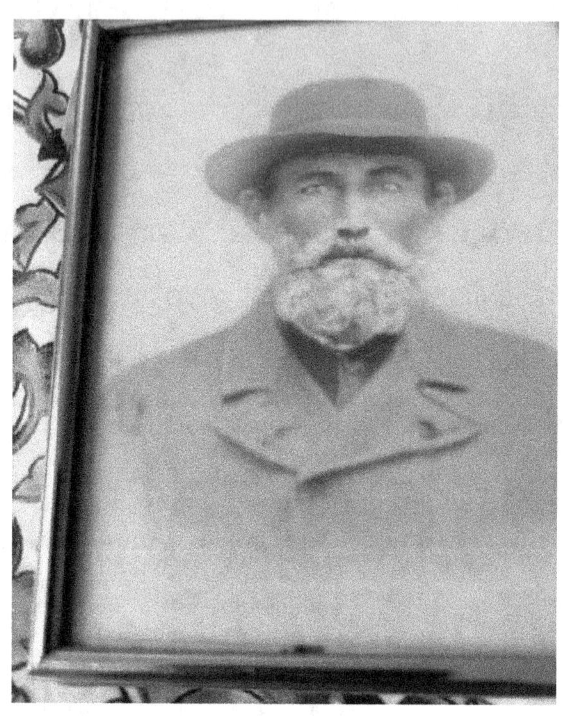

The picture which is Wolf Moskovits but labeled
on the back of the picture as Samuel Moskovits was
provided by Helen. This was said to be Wolf. Helen
admired her grandfather, Wolf, says Helen's
granddaughter Carol.

In childhood, Helen had told her granddaughter

Melinda that she was lucky to have a grandmother because Helen had never had a grandmother. This could mean that all grandmothers had passed before 1900 which was Helen's birth.

Wolf was a truck driver for a bakery, ran for mayor, and changed his name by the time of the 1869 Czechoslovakian Census to Farkus Roth. Or else since the 1930 Census reveals that Samuel Moses Roth is born in Zboj, one more possibility is Zelik Moskovits born in 1938 on the Zboj 1930 census with a son Mendely Moskovits in 1864, however Farkus means Wolf.

There is a second to the third cousin of Judith Roth, User Name Judy Jackson, who matches Lucille who is the daughter of Helen, as a second cousin. Judy was born in Cluj, Romania; her father was Martin, and her uncle was Victor Roth. They were M.D.s. That is one other clue about Romania.

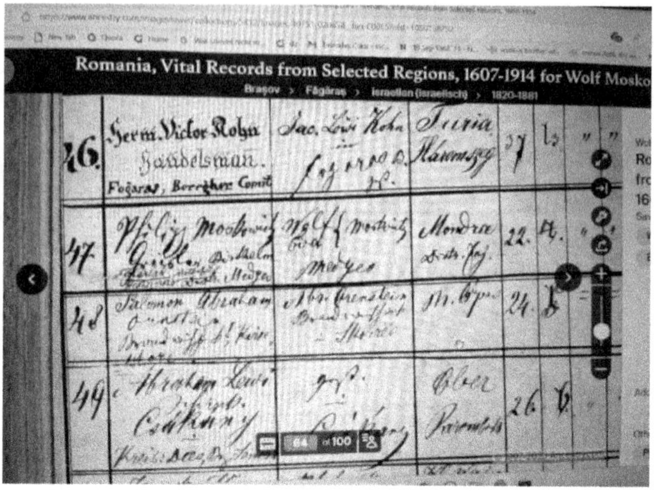

The major other clue was that Samuel Moses Roth was born in Zboj according to the 1930 Czechoslovakian census.

According to the 1869 Czechoslovakian Census for Zboj, if Samuel Moses Roth's father was indeed Farkus Roth and living in Zboj, Slovakia, as stated in the 1930 Czechoslovakian Census, then Samuel's father was originally named Wolf Moskovits. It appears that "Farkus" could be a variation or nickname for "Wolf," which seems plausible. Also, different occupying countries required changes of names. Oral testimonies from Carol, Shirley's daughter, and Lucille, Helen's daughter, and Lynn, granddaughter of Max support the existence of Wolf Moskovits within the family.

Recently, through the 1930 Czechoslovakian Census, the siblings of Helen Roth are 1) Lenka, born 1913 and living with her parents; Helena, born 1915 who was living in Sztarina with her aunt by marriage Hermina Gunczenberger. Helen born 1900 had also told of working at the tavern before she had emigrated.

Salamon born 1909 was living as a working soldier in another town; Leia, born in 1910, who is the wife of Salamon seemed to be in Humenne with Lenka later on.

Lenka, born in 1913, was the only sibling living with her parents in 1930, according to the 1930 Czechoslovakian Census. Salamon was born in 1909 and was on the Czechoslovakian Census and was a soldier stationed elsewhere, and Helena was born in

1915. Helena is not Chensche who had changed her name to Helen and was born in 1900.

Helen, born in 1900, worked at her aunt Hermina's by marriage's tavern in Sztarina. Hermina was a widow of Rifka Gunzcenberger's brother Henrik. Hermina Gunczenberger was now with her new husband, Josef Neumann. These are the siblings of Hensche who had changed her name to Helen Roth born 1900 who emigrated from Kolbasov in 1921. The siblings who had emigrated were Max, who was born in 1899 where the ship says he was 19 when he left and his granddaughter says he was 16 when he left. The ship date was 1913 which makes him 14 years of age when he went to United States.

Harry, who was born in 1892 and Lynn also said he had left at 16 years of age, although his ship date was 1907, which makes him 15 years of age; and Hensche, who was born in 1900 left at 20 in 1921.

How does a girl leave a mother for good? How

desperate does a person have to be?

The woman was a non-curious child and once did ask, "Why did you leave?"

And Helen, sitting in her husband's chair in the living room of the row home in Allentown, Pennsylvania, said, "We were very poor."

The way she pronounced the word "poor," one did not dare to ask, "How poor?"

Another time, the grandmother Helen Roth, who married a Roth, volunteered the information that she had twelve brothers who were killed.

She said this while sitting on her husband's chair in the living room of the row home in Allentown during the woman's childhood.

But recently, Vladimir, the son-in-law of Alex Roth, Jr., has discovered from the 1930 Czechoslovakian Census from the original language version that Samuel Moses Roth and Rifka

Gunczenberger had a total of nine children. Three died before World War II, three emigrated from Slovakia, and three remained in World War II- Lenka, Helena, and Salamon.

Aunt Lucille, the granddaughter Carol, and the granddaughter Lynn of Max all believe there were eight siblings of Helen born in 1900, which corroborates the 1930 Czechoslovakian Census.

The Slovak Civil Document for Births, Deaths, and Marriages available from JewishGen.Org was a requirement for citizens to register beginning in 1895. This was a recording of the people who were of Hungarian lands which were now being given back to Slovakia.

The siblings in order for Chenshe born 1900 who had changed her name to Helen are:

1. Harry (born in1892), (not on civil document). He left when he was 15 years of age. His arrival was 1907.

2. Etel (born in1896), (on civil document) (Etel marries Juda Gluck in 1938 when she was 41, both are in their 40's. Both parents of Etel are listed in 1938, so Regina Gunczenberger is probably alive since another marriage on the same list just lists a mother with no father.). Etel cannot be found on the 1930 Czechoslovakian Census.

3.Max (born in1899), The ship says he was 19 but his granddaughter says he was 14 years of age. His arrival date on the ship is 1913 which makes him 14 years of age. (According to the United States Census for 1920, Max was born in 1898, he immigrated in 1913). He is not on the civil document- he may have been born in 1894 before the civil documents began.

4. Chensche (born in 1900), (on civil

document). She emigrated in 1921.

5)Mihaly, Melech, Morris (born in1902), (on civil document). He had a heart problem and was supposed to sail.

6) Katalin (born in 1904), (on civil document).

Katalin or Katerina married Isador Bergita born in 1902. They marry in 1927 and Katerina is not alive in the 1930 Census. Katerina is listed as the daughter of Samuel Moses Roth and Rifka Gunczenberger Rothova.

In the 1930 Census Isador Bergita from Male Berezne is born in 1902 marries a woman named Gizela from Kolbasov and child Sarlota is born in 1928. This marriage happened in 1894 but perhaps the 1894 date is a mistake. Isador was from Male Berezne and he was born in 1902. Did Katerina change her name to Gizela? Later in the invasion with Salomon, a Gizela was revealed as a niece to Saloman. She may have been the seamstress.

Did Izador marry two women? His alleged grandfather with the same name had a biological daughter with Dora Morganbesser who died while giving birth to a child.

7)Salamon (born in1909), (on civil document, he marries Lina Smirlovsky in 1937). Regina Gunczenberger is apparently alive.

8)Lenka (born in1913) and (on 1930 census/not on civil document). She marries a Honig and has two daughters and lives in Humenne).

9)Helena (born 1915) and (on 1930 Census and not on civil document.)

As of the 20 of March 2024, Alan Rosenberg, whose great-great-great uncle married a Gunczenberger both of whom owned a five- and - dime store in Northampton, Pennsylvania, has pointed out a new discovery, and that is of

Chensche's three sibling names, dates, and her date from a Civil Record of Slovakia available on JewishGen.Org.

Searching for Surname (phonetically like) : ROTH AND
Any Field (contains) : ZBOJ
3 matching records found.
Run on Tue, 19 Mar 2024 21:13:14 -0600

Name	Birthplace Date of Birth Sex	Father Mother	Registration Town District County	Comments	Source Image / Record File
ROTH, Henrika / Chentse	Kolbaszo 110 F	ROTH, Samuel GUNCZENBERGER, Regina	Ulics Szinna Zemplén	Father age 36, grocer, b. Zboj. Mother age 29, b. Sztarina	SSA Humenne, Ulic Births Vol.02 003/1900-085 Ulics_Births_Vol02_003
ROTH, Mihaly / Melech	Kolbaszo 27-Mar-1902 M	ROTH, Samuel GUNCZENBERGER, Regina	Ulics Szinna Zemplén	Father age 37, smallholder, b. Zboj; Mother age 30, b. Sztarina	SSA Humenne, Ulic Births Vol.02 016/1902-059 Ulics_Births_Vol02_016
ROTH, Katalin	Kolbaszo 07-Jun-1904 F	ROTH, Samuel GRÜNCZBERGER, Regina	Ulics Szinna Zemplén	Father age 40, grocer, b. Zboj; Mother age 33, b. Sztarina	SSA Humenne, Ulic Births Vol.03 010/1904-69? Ulics_Births_Vol03_010

According to this Slovakian civil document, people of all religions, had to register for countries that had been Hungarian and had now been given back to Slovakia.

Etel was born in 1896, Chensche was born in 1900, Mihaly in 1902, and Katalin or Katerina in 1904. and Salamon was born in 1909. These names were on the civil document from JewishGen.Org and were of the time when Hungarian lands were being given back to Slovakia. This civil register began in 1895 which makes one think that Max was born before 1895 since he is not in the civil register.

Recent discoveries have also revealed the marriages of 1) Etel Roth to Juda Gluck, both in their 40's in 1938, 2) Salamon Roth to Leia Smerlovska, in their 20's in 1937 and 3) Katerina Roth to Isador Bergita who may have remarried to another woman by 1930 or Katerina could have changed her name to Gizela.

The woman is amazed that no one, including herself, asked how many siblings this woman, Chensche Roth, who was born in 1900, had.

Chensche's great niece, Lynn, said that the twelve that Helen had said that had died, were perhaps the victims of the house invasion by Bandanistas—Salamon, who was born in 1909, was there in the house invasion in 1945. In 2022, the woman and her second cousin Alex Roth, Jr. recited a prayer in front of the building of the invasion in Kolbasov. At the same time, the Ukrainian sirens were sounding. There were big, beefy guards with large rifles at the Ukrainian border that day right by Kolbasov, and Vladimir, Alex's son-in-law, was going to take the relatives with the woman across the border, but the guards did not allow this in 2022.

Erez Robinson a grandson of a survivor Helena Jacobovic of the Kolbasov invasion has translated the testimony by Survivor and Grandmother Helena Jakobovic. The translation is available on the tree of Roth/Gottlieb within Helena Jakobovic's "Gallery" of the Tree.

The details of Kolbasov in 1945 are very important and have been gleaned from the translation of the interview by Hedenka a friend and at times Helena about the invasion:

1)"There were no cars" in Kolbasov in 1945.

2)After the war, the survivors were planning to go to Snina to "buy things".

3)A seamstress was at the house in Kolbasov and was going to help sew items for the people in the house.

4)Helena Jakobovic was wearing shoes.

5)The survivors went on the roof where there was hay.

6)Schlomo or Salamun Jakobovic placed two legs in one part of the pants by accident because of nervousness.

7)There was a balcony in the house.

8)There was an apartment in Mendel Polak's house. There was liquor and food. There was a type of store there. He was a tavern owner.

9)There was a front room.

10)There were valuables of money and clothing.

11)There were 13 people in the house for six months. There were cousins and a husband and wife and Salamon Roth.

12)There were no cars-there were only carts and horses.

13)In Mendel's house there was arguing about the division of what was left there, a milking cow and a sewing machine.

15)Mendel took care of everyone. He was like a father.

16)After the war there were Jewish communities who took responsibility for the people.

17)Helena Jacobovic testified to many Jewish communities in larger villages nearby.

18)The Bandinistas allegedly who the survivor said had spoken Ukrainian were looking for Aron Teichman from Ulic who had many businesses some as the interviewer said were "shady". He hid in hay from his yard in 1945 in Ulic and later left for the United States. There was an attic with hay.

19)Mendel Polak's house was not a house with floors. This was a private one- story house. There were several rooms, a store, a grocery store, two to three stairs, a house like all in the villages. The upper storage was where the hay was. There were five rooms below.

20)They were to come with a horse- drawn cart.

21)They had intended to go to buy fabric and yarn in Snina,-that was Helena Jakobovic and sisters.

22)There was a coach.

23)The sisters walked in Kolbasov-no one had a cart and horse-they walked to Schlomo or Salamon Jacobovic's house. There was no cart and horse nor was there a cow after World War 11.

24)They were in bed in pajamas and Schlomo Jacobovic wanted to wear pants.

26)People gathered and argued about the property.

27)The custom was to bake bread on Thursday and they would make dough and they turned on the oven. This wood- fire oven was with pita bread. This was baked for the invaders and it had been intended for Friday as challah.

28)Helena said, "We baked in our house yeast dough, like pita, thick pita."

29)"Eating was in the dining room with a spicy drink," said Helena Jacobovic.

30)The Krechme had a separate entrance.

31)"They brought them from the krechma-food and eggs."

32)There was a guard of the village-he did not tell about Schlomo Jacobovic who had gone home because he wanted to be "in his bed." Helena said, that the farmers felt "solidarity because he was a farmer like them." This person, the guard, was requested to be honored by Yad Vashem.

33)Helena's uncle is Uncle Roth.

34)Helena spoke Ruthenian.

35)After Helena survived, she went to high school and worked in Prague.

36)Aron Teichman from Ulic used "to hang out" in Kolbasov; he left for the United States about a month later. He was at Schlomo Jacobovic's.

37)They did not know what happened in Ulic or they would have run away.

38)The brother of Helena was from Ruska.

39)Ruska is by the Polish border, Turnbka-Velka Profana.

40)Helen's brother lived in Okras Sanina.

41)"Eimelech Honig -he will tell me what it was in Hungarian." (Names were changed when the different countries occupied lands, similar to Wolf Moskovits to Farcus Roth.)

42)Gisela was the seamstress.

43)"And even more strange. Here Salamon Roth doesn't appear at all, you know?"

"Now?"

"He doesn't appear."

"He was everyone's boss. Yes."

"You see, he appears in Hedenka's testimony."

"Shalamon Roth. He does not appear here in the book."

"No, no (could be) and that's where, he lived this Roth." It was Gizela Krummerova's uncle. Yes. They also were from somewhere from Pooline."

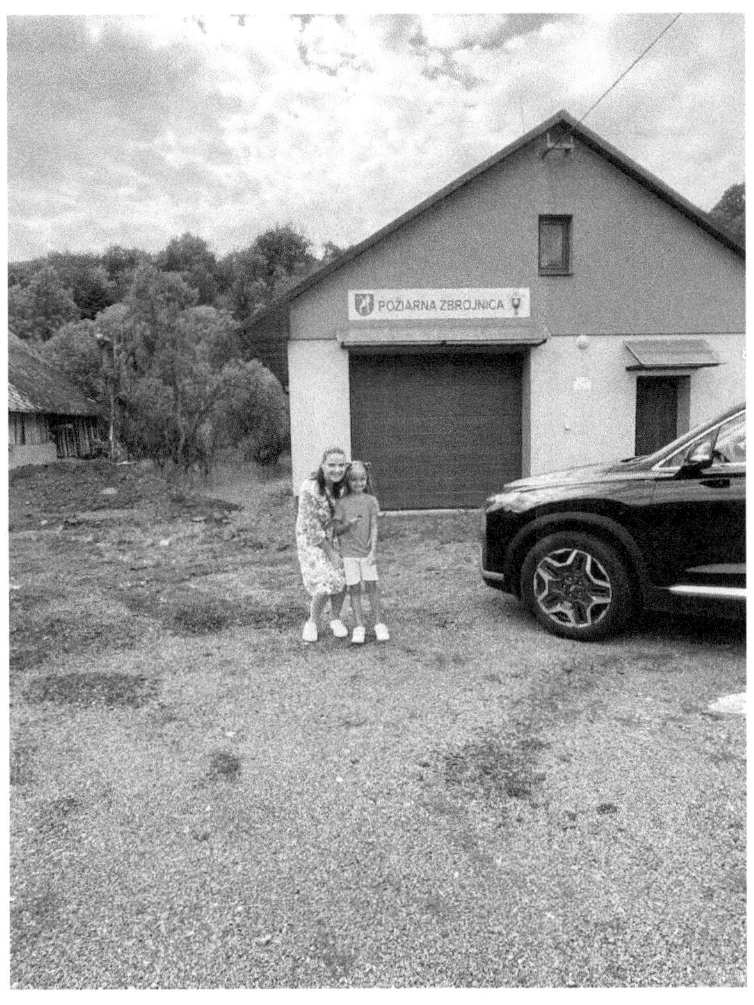

This is the Kolbasov building where the invasion took place.
Sona Rothova Buriankova the daughter and granddaughter
Klaudie of Alex Roth, Jr. were discovered by American relatives
in 2019 as descendants of the survivor Samuel Elias Roth.

44) Frieda Kessler lived with Helena in a Joint Youth House.

45)"The Hungarians came in 1938. I was only 13. Helena was younger -10 years old."

46)"Then we didn't finish primary school. Helena worked in a shop that sold hats in Prague," (after 1945).

47)Schlomo Jacobovic was the witness for Salamon's wedding in 1937.

This ends the details of the interview that help to describe what Kolbasov was like in 1945 with all due respect, the statements out of quotes have been paraphrased.

Kolbasov is made up of green, small hills with crafted cottages and is a flat land. There are rising Carpathian Mountains in the backdrop of Vysna Jablonka and nearby Kolbasov, and farming for both villages continues with people working there. The woman has checked carefully the 1930 Czechoslovakian Census in Humenne, Zboj, and

Kolbasov, and Ulic, and no Roths nor Moskovits seem to fit those years of Rifka Gunczenberger's baby-bearing years.

Researchers can press "Research" at the top, within JewishGen.Org, then the "Surname," and then next to "Data" one should press "Field" for a very small village. One can just press "Field" for a small village as well to learn all the residents of that village.

Chensche changed to Helen had four children; the surviving child said that Helen had "Gypsy boyfriends" and that Helen worked as a tavern worker in Sztarina with her mother's relatives who were Gunczenbergers. One leader in the book "The Hapsburg Jews" said that the tavern workers were called parasites by the government leaders in "The Hapsburg Jews" a non-fictional historical book, and Shirley's daughter, Carol, said that Helen worked in a tailor shop and that an aristocrat came in one day.

In Allentown, Helen made an outfit for all nine grandchildren. She used a mannikin to make the outfits. She made her own soda in a pantry room behind the kitchen. When something went wrong, she would scream out, and her neighbor would come. The neighbors belonged from different religions in Allentown. The nurse in training was not allowed to socialize with a Christian neighbor of a different sect.

There was always an entourage of men around Chensche in the 1960's in her living room in Allentown, she had vanilla cookies baking, and men were sitting around talking to her. Monro spoke of her rhubarb pie. Morris Lang or Maurice and Mr. Schneider and Herb Hyman were often there.

Once, a man spoke in Slovak on the front patio of the row home. The woman and others were amazed. Helen just shrugged.

Helen's husband, who came from Vysna

Jablonka, not far from Kolbasov, had come to Allentown, Pennsylvania.

Abe was from Vysna Jablonka, son of Rosalie Chaimovicsova Rothova and of Bernard Roth. Abe was born in 1894 according to the grave stone. Abe was the second brother to come to the United States. He came in 1910 and was brought over by his first cousins -children of Anna Chaimovicsova Nieman- Edith and Bertha Nieman.

Later, in 1923, Abe, formerly of Vysna Jablonka, now of Northampton, had a ring and two women in mind for marriage. This story was told by Adele Roth Wolensky, Joe's daughter. He went on the trolley with gloves, and the first stop he decided would be the first woman he married. He worked day and night supposedly at "Roth Brothers" and got his shave done by the barber daily and manicures in Northampton, Pennsylvania.

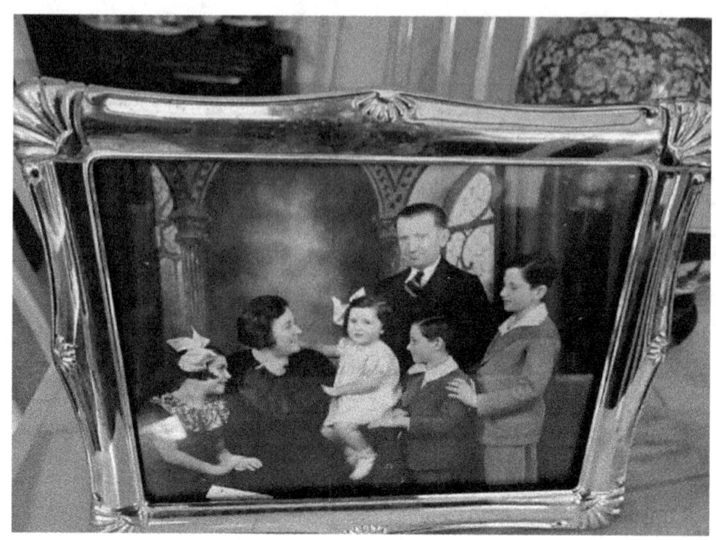

They had a maid. He worked very hard, supposedly, day and night. In 1923, when she was 23, Helen had her first baby, Monro. She always wanted to take the trolley to Allentown, and eventually, she got her wish to have a row home in Allentown on 17th St. Monro had said that he was surprised at how sensitive Helen was. According to Adele, Abe would redo the house a lot in Northampton, and Helen would go or try to go to Allentown.

Adele, the daughter of Joe, recalled that when Joe got to Allentown and had a sign on him, no one met him. Somehow Joe got to Northampton, Adele said. She remembered Phil Gunczenberger's father, Isadore, with high shoes, and Phil said you don't watch how you cross the street, and Isadore was hit by a car in New York. Isadore was the brother of Regina Gunczenberger mother to Helen Roth. When Phil went cross country, he was surprised how Adele's mother trusted him to give him money. Phil had no children and loved a waitress who took care of him at the end of his life. His brother Charles lived on a hill in a house in Northampton. Morris Lang kissed her, she said. He also was one of an entourage of visitors at Chensche's house. Tanta Chaimovics had an arranged marriage in Europe, and she ran away. Adele's mother noted that Tanta had lilly-white magnificent skin and Issy or Isador Roth and Adele's mother took care of her while Tante would switch staying at houses. Joe wore the boxes on the arms to pray -the boxes contained the biblical passages. Isador would not drive on Saturdays for the Sabbath, a holy day of rest. Meanwhile, Adele's brother Barry said that Tante had a wire hanger under her pillow and was "scary." He also said that she looked just like Rosalie Chaimovicsova Rothova in that picture. Rosalie and Tante were sisters.

As Monro was in his last months, he spoke of the war. In Tunisia, he had drinks and was driving with other men in a jeep during World War 11 in Tunisia when he yelled, "Next time in Palestine." And his Officer commanded him to get out of the jeep. The other situation was digging a hole in Northern Africa, which turned out to be a day when his mother Helen had been upset, she told Monro.

In 1924, Chensche changed to Helen had a second baby, Shirley. Helen was 24 years old, and recently, the discovery is that her name was Chensche and not Helen, and Abe was supposedly 10 years older, according to Monro, although now some documents state the age difference between Abe and Helen as seven years or six older than she was if one uses the civil Slovak record with Helen born in 1900 and Abe born in 1894 according to the cemetery. He was working day and night supposedly. In 1928, Harold was born, four years after Shirley had been born. Then, in 1932, Lucille was born.

Lucille survives.

Bernard is the father of Abe, and he remained in Vysna Jablonka. Abe, who was born in 1894, arrived in the United States in 1910; He is 16 years old when he leaves. Isador was born in 1890 and came in 1907; he is 17 when he leaves. Joe was born in 1897 and went to Allentown, Pennsylvania, in 1925 and he is 28 when he leaves. He returned in 1936 to get his sister and children and her husband, his parents, and his brother's children which were two. Samuel Elias Roth survived and created 69 people from his bond with Maria after the war.

With Abe, Abe had four children; with Isador, he had seven; and with Joe, three. Isador's love of his life was Rose Pachter, but he did not marry her until 1946. He was superstitious because his mother, Rosalie Chaimovicsova Rothova, had the same first name. He then married Rose Pachter in maybe 1946, after he had heard about the loss of his mother, Rosalie. "The love of his life" was Rose, and Isador married Rose in 1946 after his first wife, Lillie Weiss, passed in 1936 after she had given birth to seven children.

So far, there have been several incidents in 1936. The English king abdicated for love. Lillie Weiss, the wife of Isador, passed after she had seven children. Helen Roth's father passed from a natural death and had a grave placed in Kolbasov, where Melinda and Alex Roth went to that same grave in 2019. Joe Roth returned in 1936 to Vysna Jablonka and then went to Michalovce to take a picture of his family and ask them to come to the United States.

In about 1946, Rose Pachter married Isador Roth, and one child from Rose and one child from

Isador-both later married each other. Another child of Isador, was in love with this same male child of Rose but another sister had been triumphant in the love match between Rose's son and Isador's daughter.

Isador was superstitious because Rose Pachter had the first name of Isador's mother. So, he would not marry her until he had learned that his mother had passed. Rose Pachter was the love of Isador's life, Adele Roth Wolensky said.

With Jacob, son of Joshua who was brother to Bernard, there was Manny, Saul, Joan and another daughter, and a son-there are four doctors out of four children from Saul and Joan. There is Manny, who had Cheryl, and Cheryl had Lauren Weisenberger, who wrote "The Devil Wears Prada."

Of the children, one family had four; another became a doctor and had one autistic child; and another had four; he married a Catholic woman and rode the car on a Saturday, which hurt his father- one is institutionalized. Five has two daughters. Five wrote a play on Off-Broadway that explained how Isador was enamored of Helen after Isador's wife had passed away in 1936.

One daughter has two biological and two adopted, and one biological married the daughter of Bob Dylan.

Emmanuel or Manny has Cheryl, who has Lauren Weisenberger, who wrote: "Devil Wears Prada." Cheryl says that Lauren used to walk to the dinner table as she continued reading a book. Emmanuel had a child who had a developmental problem.

There seemed to be perhaps endogamy with parents who married both from Hungary or, rather, the Hapsburg Empire. The tribe and religion have been reproducing as other tribes, cultures, and religions have for hundreds of years. People were allowed to travel throughout the Hapsburg Empire until about the 1850s, according to "The History of the Hapsburg Jews."

The woman's mother's father was a psychiatrist from Hungary. This psychiatrist was violent, so Zelda raised the daughter alone,

The Gottlieb side of the woman's mother's father's side were scientists with many divorces. When the satellite went to the moon, Mimi's first cousin, Peter Gottlieb, was at the control center.

The woman's mother's father's side, Gottlieb on her father's side, and Gunczenberger on the father's mother's side make Mimi and Monro 5th to 8th cousins. Three people were tested from the woman's father's side that matched the mother's Gottlieb side, Joan Roth Lichtenstein, through Rosenbloom, Adele Roth Wolensky through Shmulkovic, and Lucille Roth Lehrich through Gunczenberger.

Mimi is related through her father to Monro's

mother's mother's side of Helen. Again, there is a lot of endogamy with people from Hungary or, rather, the Hapsburg Empire.

There is another survivor from Allentown but originally from Humenne, and Eva Levit had distant relations with Helen Roth.

Helen had two sisters and a brother, Salamon, during World War 11; three passed before World War 2-Etel, Morris or Mihaly, Katalin or Katerina; three emigrated-Helen, Max, and Harry.

Salamon was part of the house invasion in Kolbasov. There were plans to save them. Helen collapsed after the war when she saw "Life Magazine" and the pictures of the bodies. Lucille took over hanging the wash.

Helen's family's grandchild, there is one boy, and he has two boys. One boy is named Samuel, who could be like his great great maternal grandfather, Samuel Moses Roth. Samuel Moses Roth, the father of Helen, has a grave in Kolbasov and passed in 1936, and his grave states "Zev Hacohen," which means "Wolf who was a Cohen," which is a high priest; Zev Hacohen was the father of Samuel Moses Roth. Melinda Aimée Roth and Alex Roth, Jr. said the prayer at the Kolbasov cemetery in 2019 and found out later that this was his grave. A grave is the luxury.

Monro, son of Abe and Helen, worked until 91 as an English professor at Lehigh Community College. He lost a child to an illness. He had all redheads, like the Chaimovics of his father's mother's side.

Helen had a full life and went to Florida, danced in Florida, and lived there after Abe had passed. She had a gentleman friend whom she broke the heart of allegedly. Some say he ended his life. She vibrantly lived life. She had to work as a cook at the end of her life.

There was always an entourage at her house, and Herb Chaimovics, son of Elmore Chaimovics and Berta Roth, would visit and open the refrigerator.

Chensche of Kolbasov had her point of view also. Chensche was born on a pallet in her two-room house in 1900 in Kolbasov, Slovakia, from Rifka Gunczenberger and Samuel Moses Roth.

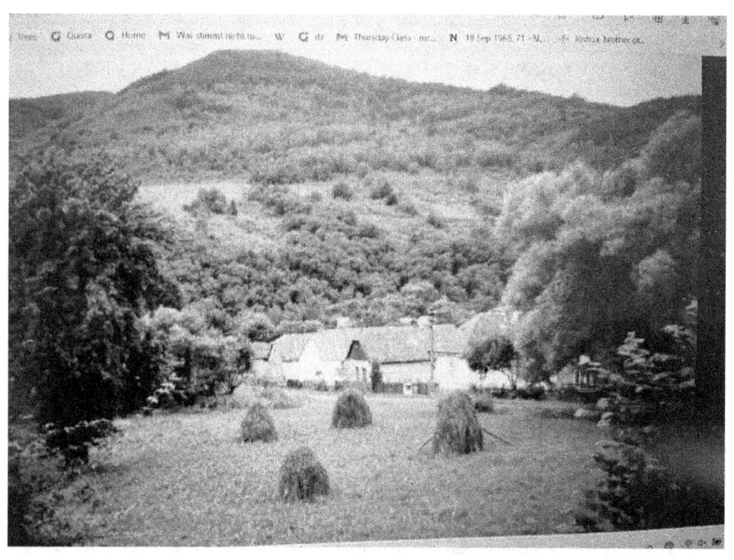

Samuel Moses Roth had been born in Zboj, a nearby village, and in 1869, the Census read that there was a Farkus Roth, who was born in 1832 and passed probably before Hensche left in 1921 for

Scranton, Pennsylvania., and a son Mosko Roth, born in 1864 and passed in 1936 according to the cemetery stone, and was Samuel Moses Roth.

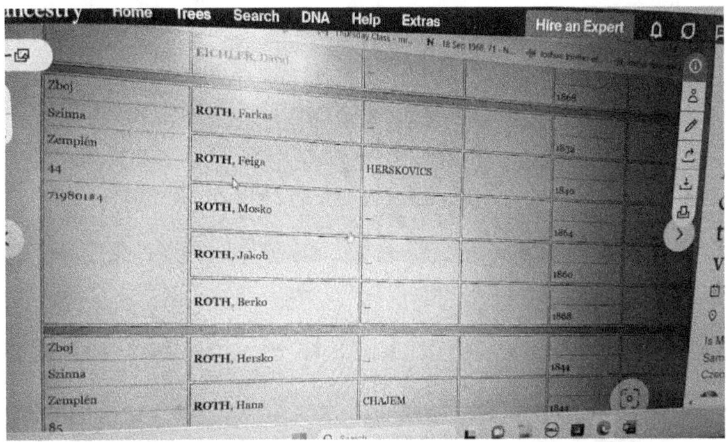

Wolf Moskovits, born in 1832, was the previous name of Farkus Roth, and Mosko was Samuel Moses Roth, who was born in 1864. In order to avoid being drafted, he changed his name.

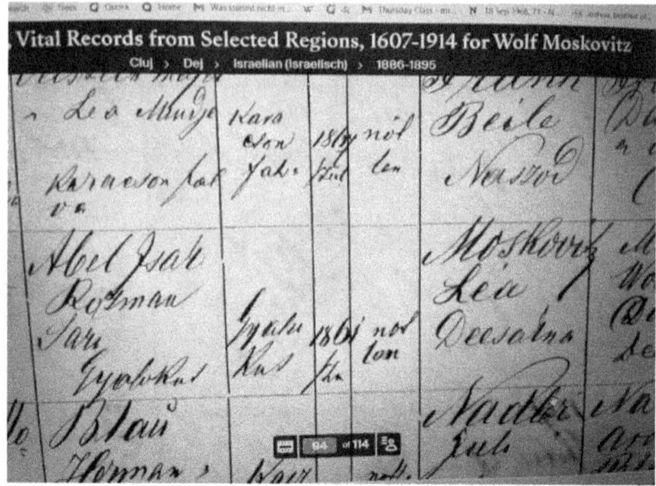

Chensche's granddaughter, who was Judith
Roth's second to third cousin, shares an identical
Deoxyribonucleic Acid of 100 Centimorgans with
Judith. Judith was born in Cluj, Romania, and the
handwritten records appeared to support Chensche's
grandfather Wolf Moskovits that he came from
Romania.

***

Wolf Moskovits, who lived from 1832 to
possibly before 1921 and, according to Chensche's
grandchild, changed his name to Roth in order to

avoid conscription-he took someone's identity, said Lynn, granddaughter of Max, and so his wife being named Rothman could make sense because many times, husbands took wives' maiden names. A handwritten census speaks of a Rothman for a wife. Wolf Moskovits was Chensche's favorite relative, said Carol, Chensche's granddaughter.

This great-great-granddaughter, Carol, mentioned that Wolf had run for mayor and worked as a truck driver for a bakery. He was also fluent in six languages.

In one census, a Wolf Moskovits was listed as a landlord in Humenne.

Chensche spent her childhood years in the two-room house where she would stay with Mother Rifka. 1)Harry born in 1892, 2) Etel in 1896, 3) Max born in 1899, 4) Chensche born in 1900, 5) Mihaly born in 1902, 6) Katalin born in 1904, and 7) Salamon born in 1909, 8) Lenka born in 1913 and 9)

Helena born in 1915.

Lenka married Yasov Honig and had two daughters. Leia, born in 1910, was the wife of Salamon born in 1909,

Max would walk three miles to school, but he would remove his shoes before setting out to protect the leather.

Mother Rifka, who lived from 1872 to possibly 1942, had Aunt Hermina as her sister-in-law. Because Hermina's husband died in World War One, Aunt Hermina had been given permission to run a tavern.

In 1915, at the age of fifteen, Chensche worked at her aunt's tavern in Sztarina.

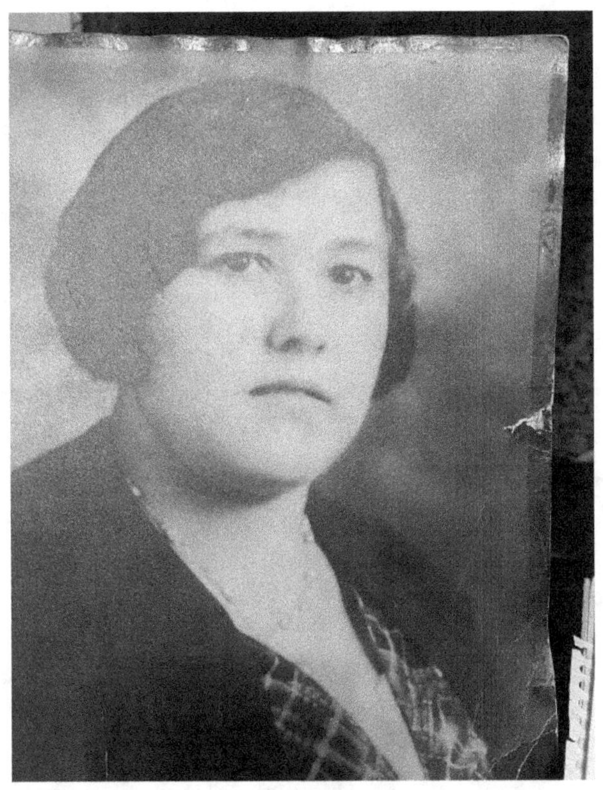

She would walk to Sztarina with her bare feet.
She had given up the idea of school because the men
and boys would stare at her darkly-set eyes, said her
daughter Lucille.

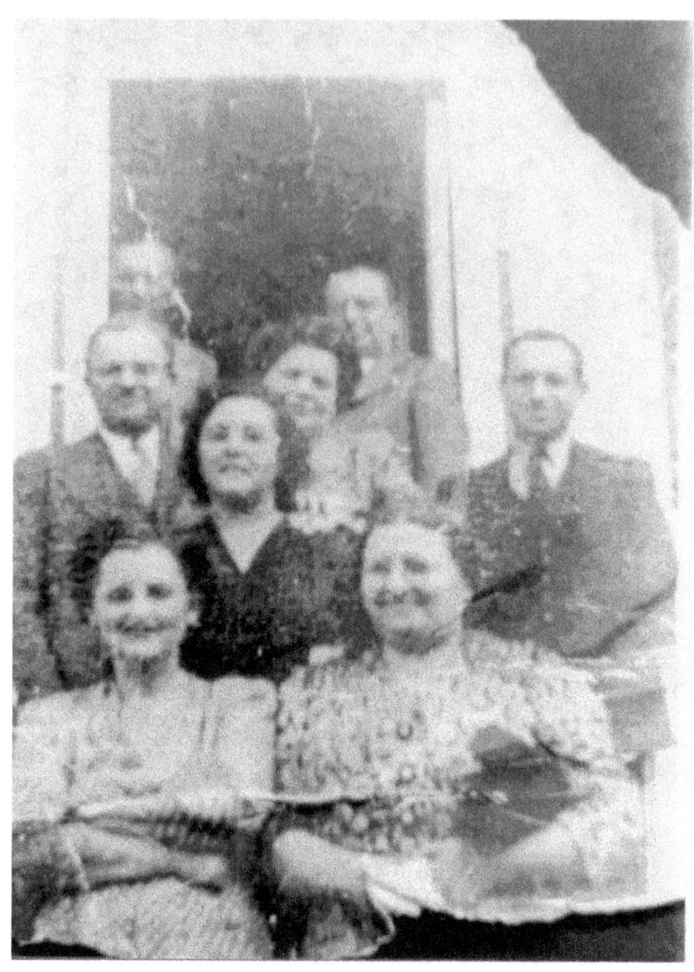

In the bottom row from left to right from the viewers' point of view are Yolan Feldman Lang and Regina Lang Roth. The second row from the bottom from left to right is Chenshe in the black dress and Joe Roth. The third row from the bottom is Isador Roth and Rose Pachter Roth. The top row from left to right from the viewers' point of view is Maurice or Morris Lang, and to the right was Abe Roth.

The woman wearing the dark dress was Chensche; she was 46 years old in 1946 when this photo was taken. Her husband Abe, born in 1894, was distantly positioned in the back row on the right side of the frame, and her brother-in-law Isador was slightly behind her.

However, in perhaps 1917, in Kolbasov, Slovakia, at the age of 17, Chenshe also proceeded to put together a plan to work in a tailor shop. One day, an Austrian Hapsburg Empire aristocrat happened to come into the business as told by her granddaughter Carol, and Chensche had then sewn an outfit for him.

Hermina Gunczenberger Neumann, Rifka's sister-in-law, was encouraging her children to leave

Sztarina, says Helena Gunczenberger Elkis. Isador, Rifka's brother, had moved to Northampton, Pennsylvania, along with Charles and Phil Gunczenberger, sons to Isador Gunczenberger and nephews of Rifka Gunczenberger Rothova. In Northampton, the hills bore eerie resemblances to the Carpathian Mountains.

There were two wood-paneled rooms in the home of Mother Rifka, who lived from 1872 to possibly 1942, with Father Samuel Moses Roth, the husband who lived from 1864 to 1936, and with Lenka, born in 1913 in the 1930 Census.

Zuzana Jedinakova's relative Jan Augusta writes and describes the houses: "All the floors were dirt and divided, usually in three or four sections. The main section was the living room with the stove, very large and made of cement or some material of that sort with a built-in chimney. . .in the winter, some people would sleep by the stove to keep warm." She adds that "a bed or two and the kitchen were in that same room." The last section, she adds, had the animals. Jan Augusta states in her four booklets of Vysna Jablonka that there are houses still like this.

In between the buildings was the Kolbasov and in Vysna Jablonka, Slovakian greenery.

However, the first two sons of Samuel Moses Roth and Rifka Gunczenberger, Harry, who was born in 1892, and Max, who was born in 1899, had started to consider leaving. In Vysna Jablonka, Jana reports in 2023 that her mother, Zuzana, who was born in 1930, Jana states that "people sowed grain, ground wheat into flour and baked bread." Jana adds that "most" of Vysna Jablonka, which Jana said was "similar" in living style to the nearby village of Kolbasov. Jana also states that "they planted potatoes, cabbage, beans, and cooked dishes from" the planted vegetables. Jana adds that the villagers had "cows, so they had milk, butter, and cheese." Isador son of Bernard from Vysna Jablonka, had his own chickens in Northampton, Pennsylvania, which is a clue that Bernard from Vysna Jablonka probably had chickens. Isador in Northampton, Pennsylvania, at first, had an outhouse for a bathroom in the 1910s. In Slovakia, Jana also adds that they had "meat for holidays" and "they made jams and fruits."

What is most important is this bit of information from Jana, daughter of Zuzana, granddaughter of Izrael Chaimovics, first cousin to Roza Chaimovicsova Roth; when Jana was asked about who was in bare feet in the village, this is what she said: "not only children but also ordinary adults walked barefoot." She continues and says, "Only on significant occasions did they wear shoes." Then, she states, "Wealthier people and their children walked around wearing shoes."

Jana also explained that "no one had a carriage in the village. Ordinary people in the village had a chariot." Yecheil's great-grandson Peter Majorovics said that people had a cart and a cow. And this unbelievable surprise that Jana reveals "Ordinary people had no free time — they worked in the fields, took care of cattle. On Sundays, they did not work; they went to church and met in the afternoons for conversations." This explanation is about Vysna Jablonka but is near Kolbasov, so Jana explains that there is a similarity. Jana, when asked what it was like for Jewish people in the village, Jana says it was the same. The only difference was whether they were poor, the Jews and non-Jews, or wealthy, with the Jews and non-Jews." Jana went on to explain that the "Jews had had their religion and their holidays" of "Shabbat... and non-Jews had their religion and their holidays."

In 1913, Max, born in 1899, son of Samuel Moses Roth and Rifka, then 14 years old, came to the United States, and Harry, born in 1892, immigrated in 1907 was 15. They left their home country at very young ages.

Chensche had several "Traveling People" as boyfriends in Slovakia, Lucille said. She also didn't attend school; according to Lucille, she instead worked at Sztarina's tavern and a tailor shop before she went on a ship to Max's home in Scranton, Pennsylvania in 1921 when she was 20 years old.

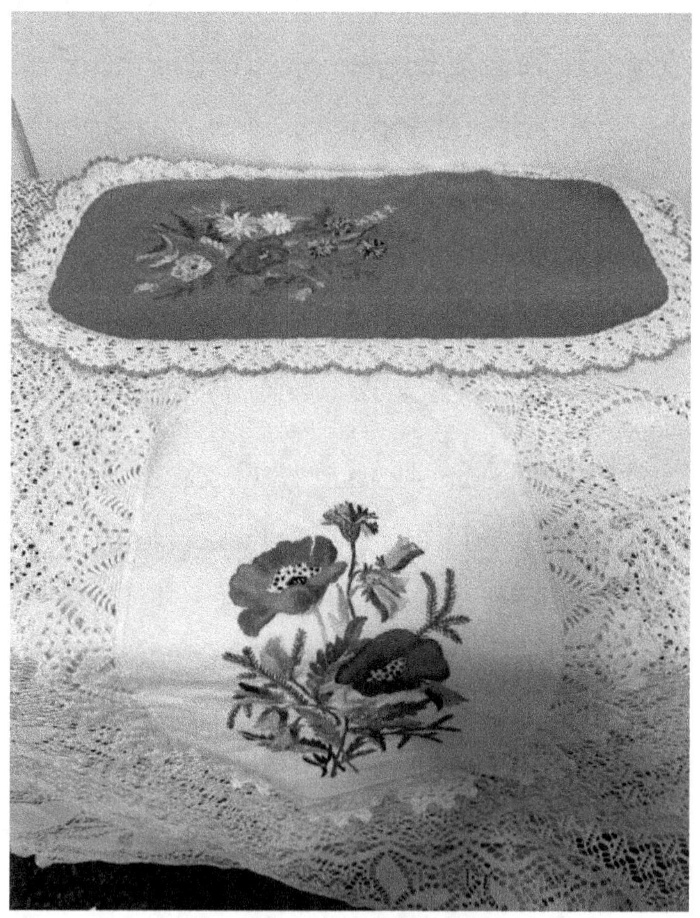

In Slovakia, according to Jan Augusta's writings on Slovakia, "every little village" had "their own peculiarities of dress…the kerchief knotted under the chin, apparently carelessly, is in reality arranged in certain folds and at a certain angle precisely as prescribed by local usage, and in a way that is different from that of the next place." Also, she adds that "the great beauty of their costumes is the embroidery, which is indeed, the chief art of the Slovak."

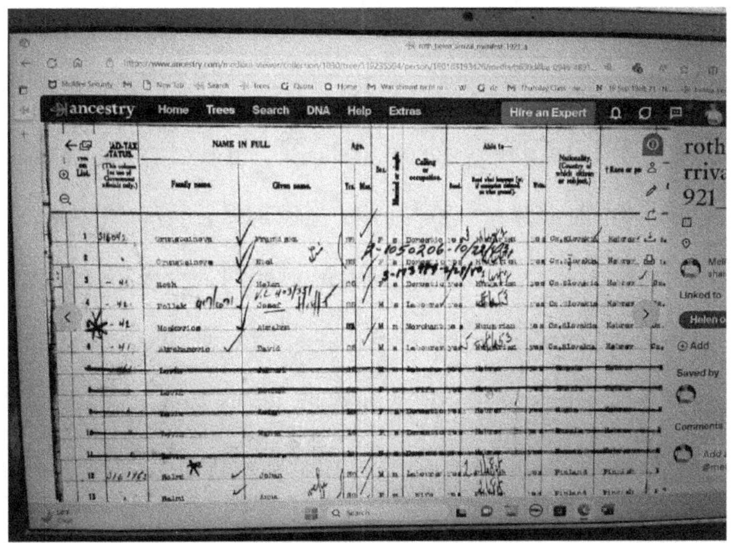

PASSENGER RECORD

Here is the record for the passenger. Click the links
on the left to see more information about this
passenger.

[ADD TO YOUR ELLIS ISLAND FILE] [VIEW ORIGINAL SHIP MANIFEST] [VIEW SHIP]

Name:	Roth, Helen
Ethnicity:	Cz. Slovakia
Place of Residence:	Kolbasoy, Cz./Slovakia
Date of Arrival:	August 30, 1921
Age on Arrival:	20y
Gender:	F
Marital Status:	S
Ship of Travel:	Olympic
Port of Departure:	Southampton, Southamptonshire, England, UK

SAVE AND PURCHASE
DOCUMENTS

View both the
original image of
the ship on which
this
passengertravelled
by clicking on the
blue buttons above
this Passenger
Record.

Chensche made a major change by Anglicizing her name to "Helen." So, a neighbor named Mr. Pollak a neighbor from Kolbasov was company along the shipping route in 1921, She cried later on in life while her son Monro was in the hospital; she asked the doctor for something for her son Monro when he discovered a relative's illness. She cried all the time after the war, her two daughters said, and she told her daughter-in-law that she must have had a bad spirit over her to get a sick child. She also cried when she saw 'Fiddler on the Roof' in New York with her daughter Shirley.

At twenty-three, although she said she was sixteen, the civil report now states that she was born in 1900, and she gave birth to her first child in America in 1923. At the age of 20, she had traveled to the United States in 1921.

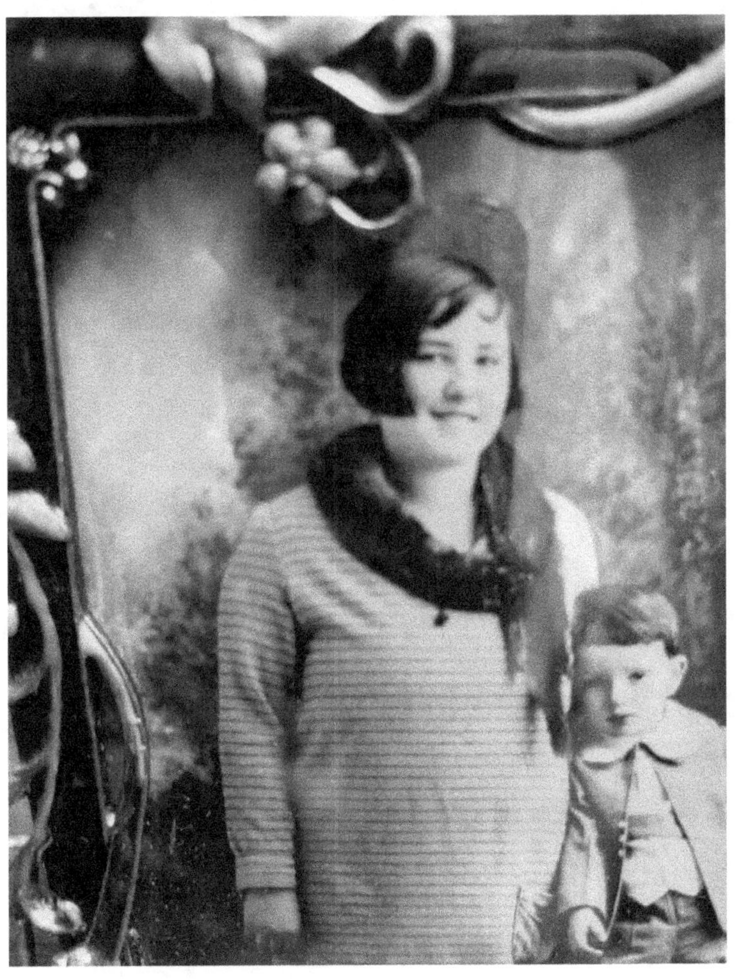

On the ship, she stated that she was 20 years old, which is in agreement with the Slovak Civil Record from JewishGen.Org.

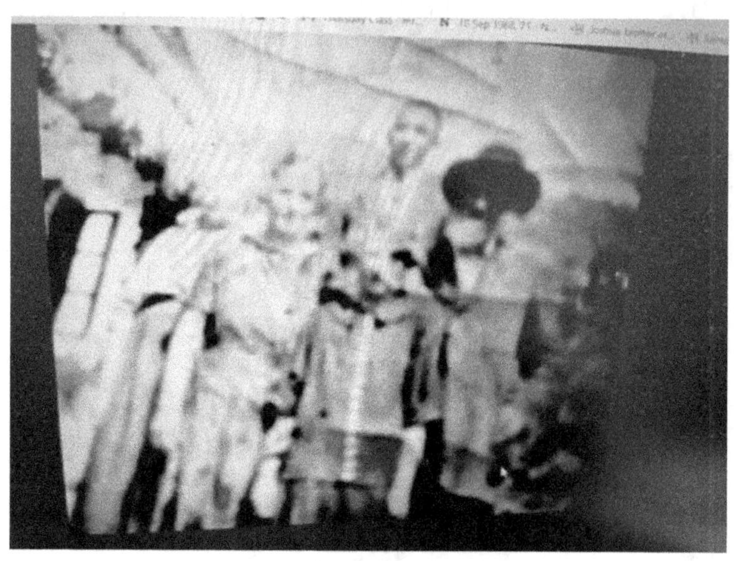

When Mother Rifka stood in front of the house, she was the tall woman in the left rear row, as seen from the viewer's view. There's a babushka- a scarf- a smiling woman with thick, attractive white hair and a grayish skirt. This is Mother Rifka. The scrawny, tall man in the back is Salamon who was born in 1909. Samuel Moses Roth, who was born in 1864, seen from the viewer's view, appears on the right. Samuel

Moses Roth has a scruffy beard and a black fedora-style hat. His wool garments were crumpled, and his mantle was not properly buttoned. The picture was possibly taken in 1930, maybe when the Census had been taken.

From the viewer's point of view, starting at the left of the bottom row, his daughter Lenka, born in 1913, is in the first row. His daughter Helena was born in 1915.

Helena, in front center, born 1915, is posing with an expression of wonder and with a horizontal crease in her frock. Lenka, born in 1913 to the left and front from the viewer's point of view, seems excited and enthralled.

Lenka, born 1913, and Helena, born 1915 from left to right first row, the sisters, years later, boarded a ship to visit Northampton, Pennsylvania, after being encouraged to see Chensche. This was remembered by Monro years later. However, the entire time they were in a house, they were separated from their parents. Later, according to Monro, the sisters sailed back to Kolbasov to rejoin their parents. Although Lucille, born in 1932, says they never came.

Lenka, on the left, was about to marry into the Honig household and go to the large city of Humenne. At the beginning of the 1940s, she, Lenka, had two daughters, Sidonia and Edita.

***

Before World War II, according to Jana Jedinakova, Zuzana's daughter and Zuzana's brother Jan who resides in Vysna Jablonka, said "Every home had a furnace for cooking," and "many had hens" and a "vegetable garden, and many made bread and jams." Jana claims that Vysna Jablonka and the neighboring settlement of Kolbasov shared "similarities," with both having students of different religions attending the primary schools. A synagogue was in Szina, and churches were in every village, she said.

In addition, the manager of Francis Shimko's DNA was interviewed about how Mary Kunso the daughter of Izrael Chaimovics and of Sofia Gula, had lived, and he told of how he had "spent a lot of time with his grandmother," and Francis stated that she was in the United States, "canning everything from the garden: lima beans, green beans, and plum," and that his grandmother who spoke Slovak "grew corn and cabbage," and "there were apple trees, peach trees, and huge grape vines or arbors," and that "cows were milked, hens provided eggs, pigs were raised and butchered: and many fish were brought home after a day of fishing." Mary Kunso came to the United States as a baby, but her "adopted" mother, Sofia Metrik, was from Vysna Jablonka and thus was probably taking on the traditions and knowledge of how people of Vysna Jablonka had lived.

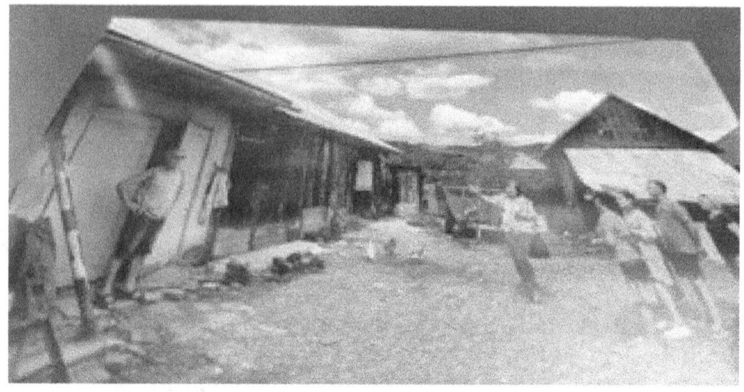

The photo is of a farm in the nearby village of Vysna Jablonka, where the fourth cousins to each other, descending from Rosalie and from Izrael Chaimovics' sides, would meet in 2019 and where Izrael Chaimovics had had relations with Sofia, Zuzana's grandmother, from this farm.

Journeyman and religious scholar Samuel Moses Roth, who was born in 1864, taught boys the customs of life's transitional rituals so they could offer prayers to God while he was walking from house to house. He also had a general store, and the census says that in addition to a total of nine children, all could read and write.

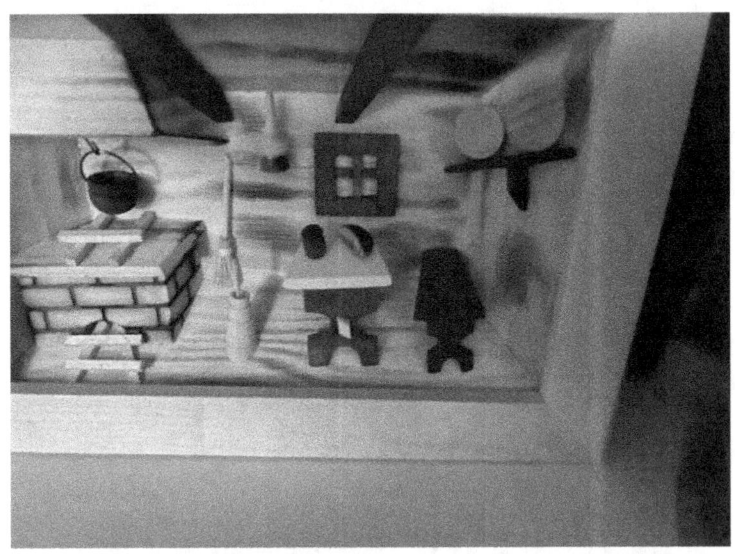

Chensche rarely attended school; instead, she would walk to the nearby big city to work in a tailor's shop. Jana, the daughter of Zuzana, who lived in Vysna Jablonka, states, "Poor and simple people grew hemp and weaved fabrics from it and sewed clothes." But there was a tailor in Kolbasov, as witnessed from the list of the 1945 invasion. One day, for Chensche, born in 1900, an aristocrat would come through the door at the tailor shop where she worked.

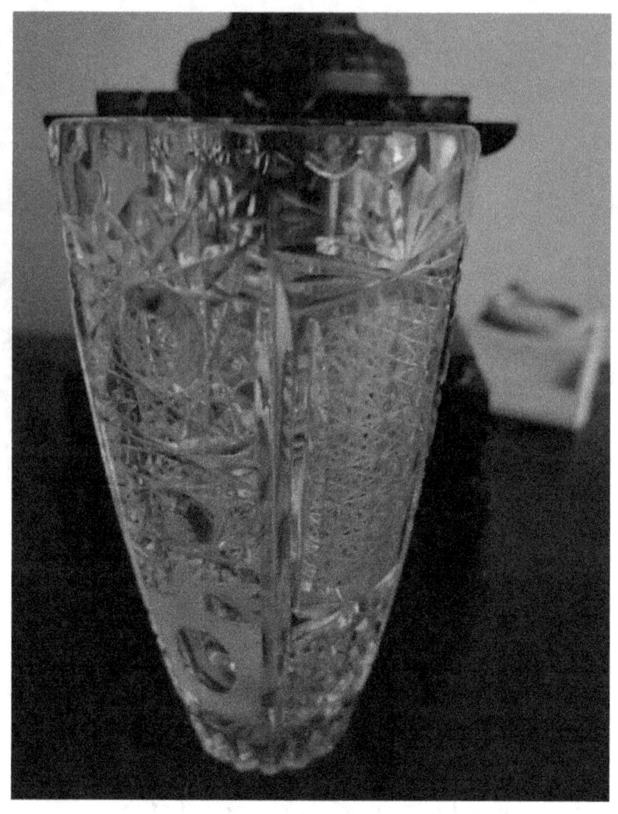

Chensche would sew the garment. Thus, she was an integral part of the Austrian Hapsburg Empire in 1917. In 1918, the country of Slovakia was no longer controlled by Hungary.

With the assistance of her parents, Samuel Moses and Rifka, Chensche accepted Hermina's invitation to work at her tavern when she was fifteen in 1915. It is assumed that since the 1930 Census, the younger Helena had been working in the tavern at 15 as well that Helen born 1900 had also worked at the tavern at 15 years old. Then, until Chenshe was seventeen years old before the Hapsburn Empire broke up, in 1917, she worked for a dressmaker and had sewed a dress for an aristocrat.. Hermina was an aunt to Chensche through marriage, and both were living in Sztarina, Slovakia, in 1915.

***

Town / District / Land	Sheet # / House # / Family #	Name / Birth Surname	Birth Date / Birth Town	Relationship	Comments	Box / Year / Reference
Kolbasov / Snina / Slovensko	0220 / 61/1	ROTH, Samuel	03-May-1864 / Zboj	head		0865 / 1930 / SNA Bratislava, Scitanie ludu 1930
	0220 / 61/1	ROTH, Regina	10-jan-1872 / Starina	wife	married 06-Jun-1888	
	0220 / 61/1	ROTH, Lenka	15-Apr-1913 / Kolbasov	daughter		
Starina / Snina / Slovensko	0299 / 27/1	NEUMANN, Jozef	12-Dec-1890 / Majdan	head		0871 / 1930 / SNA Bratislava, Scitanie ludu 1930
	0299 / 27/1	GUNCZENBERGER, Hermina	15-Dec-1892 / Ricska	partner	[previously] married 10-Jan-1911, widowed 24-Jun-1916	
	0299 / 27/1	ROTH, Helena	05-Apr-1915 / Kolbasov	relative		
	0299 / 27/1	GUNCZENBERGER, Henrich	15-Jan-1913 / Starina	stepson		
Spisska Nova Ves / Spisska Nova Ves / Slovensko	0481 / 517/43	ROTH, Salamon	22-Feb-1909 / Kolbasov	soldier	permanent address Kolbasov	1078 / 1930 / SNA Bratislava, Scitanie ludu 1930

Later, in the 1930 Czechoslovakian Census, Helena born in 1915, Chensche's sister, would work for Aunt Hermina at her tavern.

Chensche left for America in 1921 but did not attend school. Hence, the lack of letters was nonexistent for her American relatives. Thus, there was a lack of an epistolary relationship in the future of time. Rather, she worked in the tavern. She had "boyfriends," she had told her daughter Lucille years later, and they were the people who had been expelled from India, "The Traveling People," who were part of Slovakia.

In 2019, when the woman went to Teplice, Czech Republic, to stay with Alex Jr.'s family, there were "Traveling People" outside of the high rise and in the park in Humenne. There were "Traveling People" viewing a concert, and their dress was American hip-hop fashion. While in Michalovce in 2022 for the Solpierstein service, ten-year-old girls were later going from trash can to trash can and collecting soda cans. And yet the town seemed to be scrubbed neatly, and the two little girls also seemed neat and organized. That is a contrast to Frankford, Philadelphia, where the woman went in 2022 where behind Michael's row home, there were many discarded beer bottles, and his red beard was like Rumpelstiltskin as he sat on the 1800s porch and spoke to the woman in 2022, with his long beard - half red and half gray.

There is an area where many "Traveling People" live in Slovakia, and there is work. The mayor of Michalovce spoke to the woman about how the city has aided the life of the "Travelers."

Aunt Hermina, who now had a new husband, Mr. Neuman, by the time of the 1930 Census, was encouraging her children to emigrate, according to Helene Elkus, granddaughter of Hermina Gunczenberger. The sister of Abe Roth's mother, Anna Chaimovicsova Nieman, claimed years later that there was a rumor that America was "paved with gold."

****

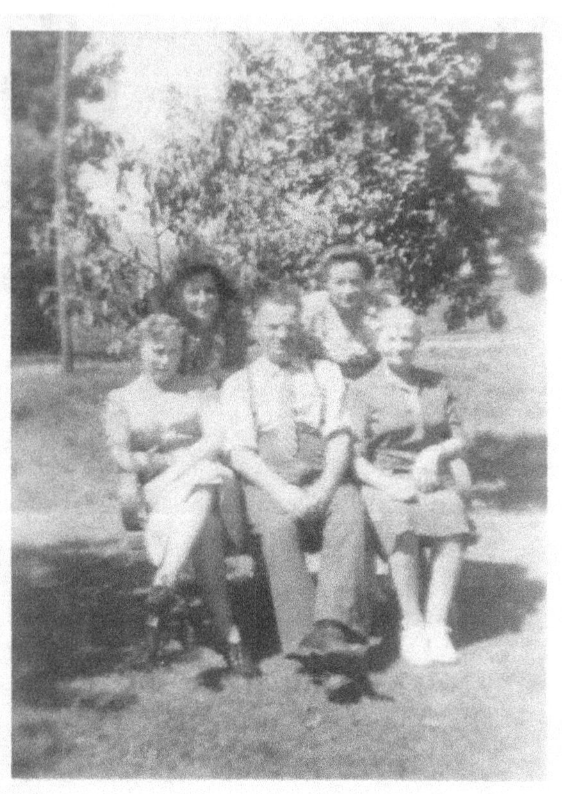

In the picture in Northampton, Pennsylvania, above from the viewer's point of view, there is Bertha Nieman on the left, Isador Roth in the middle, and Anna Chaimovicsova Nieman, sister of Rosalie Chaimovicsova Rothova, in the first row.

Sadly, Edith and Bertha would tease Tante, who wore black, and chant, "Old lady, old lady, fell in a pit," Lucille said. Tanta is not in the picture. The second row from the viewer's point of view is Isador's daughter, Henrietta Roth, on the left on the top row, and Edith Nieman on the right on the top row from the viewer's point of view in Northampton, Pennsylvania. Edith and Bertha were daughters of Anna. They had gone to Slovakia to get Abe in 1910 when Abe was 16 if he were born in 1894 which is what the cemetery stone says. The picture was taken in the late 1930s in Northampton.

Anne Chaimovicsova Nieman had worked as a maid, as told to her daughters Edith and Bertha, and as told by Edith and Bertha to the woman in the 1970s. Edith and Bertha worked at Lomans in New York City and would bring clothes for Helen, and Helen feared them because they would examine the house for cleanliness, Lucille said. Anna was the sister of Abe's mother; from the viewer's point of view, on the right of the bottom row. she had been born in

Melinda Aimée Roth

Parivoche, Slovakia.

In the meantime, the resilient mother, Rifka Chaimovicsova Rothova, was occupied with giving birth in the cottage. Harry was her first child, born in 1892. Etel was born in 1896. Max was born in 1899. Chensche followed in 1900; Mihaly or Morris in 1902, Katalin or Katerina in 1904; Salamon was born in 1909; Lenka followed in 1913. and Helena in 1915 and -nine total as the 1930 Census in the original language states. Rifka would have been too old to have more babies at 58 years of age in 1930.

Searching for Surname (phonetically like) : ROTH AND
Any Field (contains) : ZBOJ
3 matching records found.
Run on Tue, 19 Mar 2024 21:13:14 -0600

Name	Birthplace / Date of Birth / Sex	Father / Mother	Registration Town / District / County	Comments	Source Image / Record / File
ROTH, Henrika / Chentse	Kolbaszo / 110 / F	ROTH, Samuel / GUNCZENBERGER, Regina	Ulics / Szinna / Zemplén	Father age 36, grocer, b. Zboj; Mother age 29, b. Sztarina	SSA Humenne, Ulic Births Vol 09 / 003/1900-085 / Ulici_Births_Vol09_003
ROTH, Mihaly / Melech	Kolbaszo / 27-Mar-1902 / M	ROTH, Samuel / GUNCZENBERGER, Regina	Ulics / Szinna / Zemplén	Father age 37, smallholder, b. Zboj; Mother age 30, b. Sztarina	SSA Humenne, Ulic Births Vol 02 / 016/1902-052 / Ulics_Births_Vol02_016
ROTH, Katalin	Kolbaszo / 07-Jan-1904 / F	ROTH, Samuel / GRÜNCZBERGER, Regina	Ulics / Szinna / Zemplén	Father age 40, grocer, b. Zboj; Mother age 32, b. Sztarina	SSA Humenne, Ulic Births Vol 07 / 010/1904-037 / Ulics_Births_Vol07_010

Max, born in 1899, used to walk three miles to

school. He refused to wear shoes because he believed the leather would eventually wear out, Lynn, his granddaughter, said.

Max would later tell his granddaughter Lynn that he had "come steerage" because there was "nothing lower" and that he understood numerous languages because "the borders kept changing."

Harry, Max, and Chenshe went to the United States. They all traveled to Pennsylvania, where Isador Gunczenberger lived in Northampton. Max and Harry settled in Scranton, Pennsylvania.

The mayor of Humenne was in love with Chensche, Chensche's daughter Shirley said. Lucille, her daughter, mentioned that her dark-set eyes caused men to look at her. The dwelling had two rooms, maybe a hard pallet, and, as she would later remark, "We were so poor."

One day in 1921, she decided at 20 years of age that she would be leaving. She was sad to leave her mother and father, Lucille had said. Chensche left from Prague, Lucille said; she had numbness to block out her sentiments then perhaps. Chensche had taken a train to Prague, Lucille had said.

Thus, when she was 20 years old, she stated she was 20 years old on a ship bound for the United States. She noticed people on that ship eating something she had never seen before—sandwiches, as she subsequently discovered and told her granddaughter Carol about that later. They had been named after an English aristocrat, Lord Sandwiche.

At 20 years old, she came to New York and was met by her maternal uncle, Isador Gunczenberger, who then took her to Scranton, where she could see her brother Max. She then moved to Northampton, Pennsylvania, where Isadore Gunczenberger was living with a Rosenberg, and she found out about a furniture store called "Roth Brothers."

She heard that the brothers Abe, Joe, and Isador were from a village in Slovakia called Vysna Jablonka, which was close to her village, Kolbasov. Later on, in New York, she would go to a play of "Fiddler on the Roof," which was with Shirley and Carol. She understood the Yiddish, which reminded her of her Slovakian village.

So now, she walked to that store in Northampton in 1923 and got into a Slovakian conversation with Abe, and lo and behold, they were not related, but Abe began to fancy her. Abe was supposedly ten years older, but now documents state a three-year difference. One might agree that Abe was born in 1894 due to the cemetery stone and that he could not be born in 1896 which is what his date would be if the 1930 Census were accurate-he was 34 in 1930 which would make him born in 1896. That would make him four years older than Chensche.

Abe was doing well; he supposedly worked hard

at the store, got a shave at the barbershop daily, received manicures, used a handkerchief daily to open a train door, and was determined to keep doing well. One brother's son, Barry, said he gambled, had women, and took money out of the business, which was a surprise, and shockingly took life insurance policies out on his parents. Zelda had seen him with a woman at the New York train station. Brother Joe must have missed their mother, for he returned in 1936, and Isador-he refrained from marrying the woman of his life until 1946 because of his superstition of the fact that the mother, Rosalie Chaimovicsova Rothova, had the same first name as Rose Pachter.

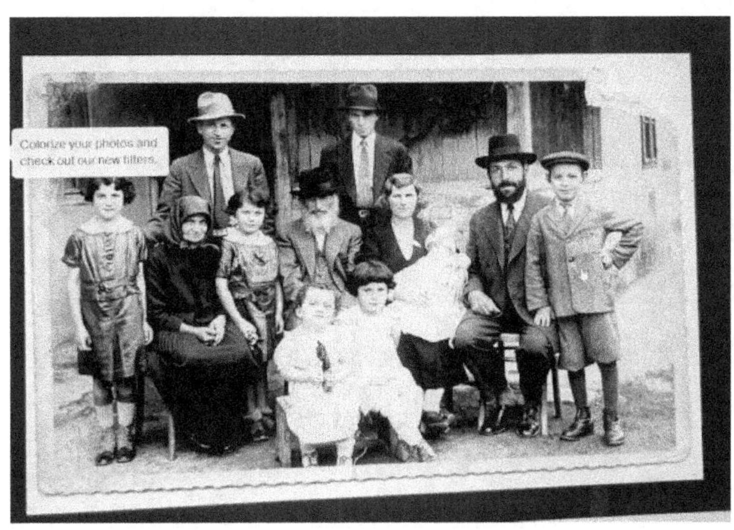

Bernard is in the picture with the white beard, and Rosalie is on the left side from the viewers' point of view and wears a scarf. In Allentown, Pennsylvania, Joe, Isador, and Abe sent money to Vysna Jablonka, and Isador refused to wed the "woman of his life," until 1946 as Joe's daughter Adele referred to her. Isador wed Lillie Weiss instead.

Isador became a widower in 1936, and he still delayed until 1946 marrying Rose Pachter. Rose would eventually become his wife, but for the time being, Isador could not wed her as Rose shared the same first name as his mother, Rosalie.

One day in 1923, Abe decided to marry and purchased a diamond ring, but he had two women in mind. Not knowing whom to propose to, he decided to board a trolley; he'd marry whoever's stop for their residence came first… The first stop was where Chensche resided, so he proposed to Chensche.

And so, he asked her… one pluck of coincidence… one weird quirk of fate… the first stop of a traveling trolley in America brought together two people from nearby villages within Slovakia.

Harold, Chensche's son, would have a son named Alan, who would have sons named Jacob and Samuel. The names were important: Jakub, the brother of Abe who had passed, had a ticket that was given to a member of Chensche's family-Chensche's brother. On Abe's side, Jakub would have a son who would survive Auschwitz and be found by American relatives in 2019. Samuel was Chensche's father, and Sofia, Harold's daughter's daughter, was also the woman who had a liaison with the first cousin of Rosalie, the mother of Abe, Isador, Joe, Jakub, and Berta. Sofia was the name of Harold's daughter's daughter. Sofia had the liaison with Rosalie Chaimovicsova Rothova's first cousin Izrael Chaimovics in 1896 and in 1900 and then another discovery of another child and then...

***

1936 was when the death of Lillie occurred, Isador's wife; the burial of Chensche's father; Joe traveling to Vysna Jablonka to try to convince his family to immigrate to the United States, and they refused; in 1936, there also was the abdication of the King of England due to "love." And Mimi Florence Gottlieb Roth, in 1936, had been instructed to bow before the principal of her New York City school. Her maternal aunt Estelle was ill in 1936 with rheumatic fever.

In 1936, Chensche traveled to now-widower Isador's house in Northampton, Pennsylvania, and another of Rosalie's sisters from Vysna Jablonka Tanta Hannah Chaimovicsova had immigrated to take care of the seven children. Chensche began to make clothes and bring food. Tanta Hannah would wear black and walk the streets.

In the play written by Beatrice Roth who
was the older daughter of the seven children of
Isador Roth, Beatrice who left at 17 years old
and who had cared for her siblings after 1936,
wrote in her exquisite play on "Off-Broadway"
from New York City with permission from the
family. "THE FATHER "(Beatrice Roth's
Play)

"He thought she would never actually leave home.
Yet when she did he visited arriving early on the
Sunday
excursion
in time to take her out to a hot breakfast.
The father believed in hot cereal.
She believed in chance," Beatrice wrote in her play.

She continued and described the exquisite mystery of
the religion. "For years after she left the father's house
she wakened still to the echo of his dovening
the father prayed an hour and a half each
his totality wrapped in stripe and fringe

his forehead strapped in leather ribbon
his consciousness trapped in holy cube containing
sacred
parchment
covering his third eye," Beatrice Roth wrote.

Beatrice continued to describe his loss and his
comfort from his spirituality in Northampton. "He
fed the pet canary while he dovened.
His murmur-song-secrets with his God seep into
their final
dream-state.
Woke and washed tumbling to their breakfast all that
remaining was the cold air from the open-and-shut
of his departure."

Isador's hard work was palpable, as she writes about
the constant work and praying and then the sudden
loss, for Isador and the seven children:

"Working early   working late
dinner was at noon everyone walked home he
gulped his food and washed his mouth and rushed
back to the store
head a-tilt
arms a-swing   unevenly
favoring the work-worn topography of his frame

was tall and dark and disappearing
his presence in the house a rarity   a scarcity
his absence a stern
turning on the Sabbath fleshly
fingers dipping honey
thawing all the week's denials," this was the imagery
of Isador in his loss and comfort.

"His teeth were small and perfect
he had them all upon his death
of course he was only sixty when he died
still in those days if you had all your teeth at sixty...

He wore a half-smile always when he dovened
that is how she came to memorize his teeth.
His intimacy was with his God.
It was the only intimacy discernible until
one day on a Sabbath as it happened
she was summoned
running in the corridor rounding the square corner
entering standing watching waiting
in her strides fresh from synagogue
his gaze bent on the silken maze
he bends
and with practiced certainty
cups and kisses
drinking drowning flooding every bone and hollow
natural so natural

the shock is thunderous.
In the corner
in the shadows
in her dark and watchful cornea
lightning strikes splitting vision
illumining
something ontological
no such fissure in her
claustrophobic
distance
with the mother
Bent above the open pine box
his arms about the tiny brothers
peppering the powdery gravel
he is sprinkling on the purpling cheeks
burying with her
in the ground
their secret," Beatrice
wrote.
And yet it was her love of life, Beatrice's and
Chenshe's which really 'took the cake' and the 'garb'
and the 'glory':

"I loved the high holidays because of the clothes.
Everybody got a new outfit. From top to bottom.
From inside to out. Everybody. Except my Aunt
Helen.
My Aunt Helen got three new outfits and on the first

day of Rosh Hashonah she appeared in her most spectacular one. My Aunt Helen was a buxom woman. She loved to sit in the front row of the balcony. She drew her chair up close to the bannister- raised her entire upper self on to it and rested there." Beatrice Roth wrote in her play, "The Trilogy."

This Off Broadway play by Beatrice Roth was performed in 1985 and was called, "Trilogy." One part of the "Trilogy" was "Seventeen," and in a brilliant excerpt, Beatrice Roth, daughter of Isador Roth and Lillie Weiss who had passed in 1936, describes this loss: And yet Beatrice reveals many solutions to many mysteries. Here, Chenshe is being described as she visited Isador and the seven motherless children in Northampton, Pennsylvania, in 1936:

"When the mother died, the father broke down and became sensual," Beatrice Roth writes in her play "The Trilogy."

Beatrice Roth continues with her play and describes a seductive woman.

"She sits.

Melinda Aimée Roth

First with headaches
                    skipping days at the
                    store
            then with touching
                    his hands uncurled
            then with softening
                    his face fell
                    into curves
        he fell
        in love
                    with his brother's wife
        She may have loved him too.
        She may have loved him all along.
                    Sure.
Vain though she was it was not all vanity responding
                    to his affection.
                            Firstly she came on.
She came on cooking serving until things could settle
                    she was warm
                    compassionate
                    there
she preferred being there her husband Abraham and
    she were not affectionate that anyone could see
    Abraham was brusque proud of her she was good-
    looking," Beatrice Roth writes in "The Trilogy," an
    Off Broadway play in 1985:
                            "Being fat was no
                            deterrent

                        those days in their
                             culture
                          being thin was
                            somewhat
                             suspect
              not having enough
            not having eaten enough perhaps

       The youngest sisters part and comb his hair.
        They hover giggle fuss and joke with him.
           He touches women in their presence
          arm about leaning in hair mingling
              this could be a comfort
                                a relief
          a girl of seventeen full of her own sense
                               and incense
                her own pursuits
                 on the bring
                               Go
                             Plunge
                            …oh…
       She breaths a path around the rim circumventing
      choosing pink ground clasping red flowers to her
                             belly
                            swaying slending
           up against the satin cutting board

stuffing tarts
fashioning Daddy's darling favorite honey cake
chopping daydreams with the onions
grinding passion with the pepper
paring jealousy wafer thin with the
stainless steel stiletto
stealing to the castle to the portals
of her unsuspecting fairy princess
pointing
jabbing
stabbing
to her very corsets staining
her *own* ardent ad rebellious landscape.   No
this is not a movie
Her *own* ardent and rebellious and o
bedient
puritan
waspish jewish
Cinderella."
Beatrice writes in her
play. The figurative
language of bathos,
pathetic fallacy, and
violent imagery as she
watched her father is
breathtakingly brilliant.

But after she had witnessed Isador, her father, she
had her reasons for leaving. She had dreams, she
knew that others were now taking care of her
siblings, but her anguish as this seventeen-year-old
wanted to leave and become an actress and leave her
father and her siblings again exquisitely these words
sort of scream out in anguish:
"He thought she would never actually
                                    leave home
              Yet when she did
                              he came to her
                              performance
         Following one as Joan
                              of Arc
         Concerned
                         she asked him
              Daddy
how was it seeing me wear a cross on my knees to
              saints and deities,"

Oh, how tender did Beatrice Roth question her
father about whether he were offended at her playing
another type of part with another religion, and how

Isador explained in such sage-like advice of the elders
of all wise religions.

"he himself did not
revere
she watched him
think watched his heart bend toward her
at last he spoke," Beatrice writes in her play in 1985 in
"The Trilogy."

In the play, Beatrice has her father wisely answering
Beatrice, "But that was Joan's belief
was it not…"

Beatrice Roth's mind was so inquisitive after having
lost her mother and after leaving home in anguish,
she writes in her play, bravely,
"I want to know you.
How you survived your birth found food how you
multiplied stood up to your first there-is-no-turning-
back
how you recognized your enemies

how you surpassed your melancholy," Beatrice
writes in the play.

Her loss of her mother and father was the stuff of
ages as she screams through brilliant words,

"In a strange bed in a hospital in a strange city
brought for one of medicine's more arrogant
experiments
the vigil with him."
"One August afternoon," Beatrice Roth continues in
her play, "Trilogy," "she and he alone receive a local
rabbi sent for to say Tilim with him. The rabbi stands
beside the bed small next to the outstretched fingers
held rigid by a needle conducting glucose through a
transparent tube attached to a pouch above the bed.
The rabbi stands
a stranger here to perform an act of intimacy.
The father's smile quavers firmly
to put the stranger at his ease.
It goes unanswered.
The glucose persists shimmying downward pressing
the reluctant vein.
The litany begins.

The rabbi's voice is thin.
The father's unwavering in its wavering.
The rabbi's words inaudible, eyes lidded by
embarrassment.
The father bypasses this licensed emissary
his voice a feather each strand articulate faintness.
Suddenly the transparent tube shudders.
The glucose shimmies backward up the tube defying
gravity.
That other tube leading from a fading intellect is lit by
a beam begun aeons earlier—a flash so dazzling, the
vein spits the unnatural fluid," Beatrice Roth writes,"
"back into its desperate channel.
The father's eyes burn black.
Singed by a current
propelling his spirit.

Days later hurried break for sandwich luncheon
detained by table service busy harassed waitress
brother-in-law chiding sister for her sadness
rush back stand a moment in the doorway
he is asleep.
One step takes you to his side.
Kiss his forehead.
It is warm

remains warm for
your kiss
though he is far
beyond
Bent over
your brother stands sobbing in the bathroom.
Bent over
your brother is bleeding on a Korean field," she
writes now about her brother Joel.

She describes the lushness of the temple in the 1930s.
"On holy days and on the Sabbath he reclined at
table and while chanting the after-dinner gratitude he
scraped and gathered every crumb and morsel until
his place became immaculate. Next morning
wrapped in stripe and fringe depending on the
weather" and then Beatrice describes his compassion
for the fauna:

"He flung wide the screen or raised the pane a crack
to scatter last night's breadcrumbs among the
gathered, feathered congregation. Of all that I recall I
sometimes think this may be what I miss most."

In the 1930s, Beatrice now describes the weather and the practice of medicine with one doctor:

"In February we had the worst blizzard in anybody's recollection. In those days Spring came in March. So February was much too late for heavy snow. That Sunday everyone stood and talked about the weather. My mother stood that Sunday in the soaking ground at old man Flom's funeral and on Monday she could not stand. Old Dr. Miller stood in our kitchen.

'Wal it's just the grippe,'

"The grippe is a very bad cold a mild flu. All that week and the following Monday old Dr. Miller stood in our parlor," Dr. Miller was the uncle of Adele Roth Wolensky and Barry Roth, Adele's brother called Dr. Miller, "The man of my life." Dr. Miller who never married was very generous to his nephews and would pay them 20 dollars to wash his car on weekends," Barry Roth described.

Beatrice Roth's play continued, "I say it's just the grippe."'

"But on Thursday the ambulance stood" "Haff Hospital. On Saturday I stood at my Saturday-after-school job when my Aunt Helen came through the door, I woke at six my sisters still asleep beside me. There was someone in the house I could hear them. They were coming up the stairs. It was my Aunt Helen. She was wearing her soft brown wool with rose-beige flecks," Beatrice writes in this mystical, supernatural feeling of various saviors at the door.

"She stood in the doorway," Beatrice continues. "I started out of bed. She started into the room. She was walking toward me. Suddenly she stopped. . .

My bobby pins stuck in my Aunt Helen's soft brown wool with the rose-beige flecks.

Embarrassed to be seen with bobby pins in my hair.

Ashamed I've been putting my hair in bobby
pins while my mother was dying. . .

That was March the second.

All of March April May June the rest of my
Senior year

My Aunt Helen cooked dinner for us

Dinner was at noon

Everyone walked home," Beatrice writes.

Oh, oh, oh, the woman now recalls Chenshe
and how she had appeared in 1972 and tried to help
and the woman's cautions. . . and then Beatrice in her
play "The Trilogy," even describes what life is like for
the rural children of Northampton, Pennsylvania:

"Except for the deep country kids who came on
the bus.

When we left in the morning it was bleak and

chill

No matter what the weather

But when we returned at noon

the house had turned to gold

There were new spring potatoes

My Aunt Helen's face was steaming above the

new spring potatoes

steaming in their jackets

The sweet butter was rolling and melting and rolling and the coarse salt was falling and falling and the sweet steaming face of my Aunt Helen spring potato salt face of my Aunt Helen..." Beatrice writes in her play, "The Trilogy." Chenshe is the woman's grandmother and to hear the description of this woman is tantalizing and shocking and magnificent.

The woman is realizing the seductive literature:

"Then she would rush to the cupboard and take down a dish of strudel dough. And when she had time to make that strudel dough I don't know because, at eight A.M. when everyone left for school and work, she was not about to start cooking and cleaning. Oh no there was the milkman

and the iceman

and the postman

and the butcher delivery," Beatrice writes. What wonderful detail about how life was with the tradesmen in the 1930s in a small Northampton town which had fame due to buried calcium carbonate that was able to be the building bricks for bridges, for the Panama Canal, and finally in Northampton, General Trexler would build a trolley car which Chenshe, the woman's grandmother, Beatrice's Aunt Helen, Helen would finally be able to go to Allentown each day by trolley from Northampton to Allentown.

But Beatrice continues,

"and Morris Lange stopping by for a chat," oh, oh, oh, this was the man who tried to follow Chenshe to the bathroom, who kissed Adele at sixteen and was seen at Cedar Park not quite covered.

But Beatrice continues to write, "and Nat Weiss coming in for advice," this is in the 1930s and Nat had a famous son who was a poet… Ted. He passed on a horse in 1945 after Chenshe had collapsed after seeing "Life Magazine" after the bodies from the war were shown with pictures from Slovakia and Nat Weiss was…

"Nevertheless, there was the strudel dough all stretched out full of holes but the most delicious pastry,":

Beatrice continues to write in an inimitable description of a woman baking pie:

"you ever tasted oh the sour-cherry strudel and the apple strudel with the cardamon and All American Spice the most exotic of all was the cabbage strudel and when she had time to shred that cabbage so perfectly and marinade it so perfectly with those perfectly browned onions I don't know but there it was six o'clock all rolled oiled oven-ready and not a spot on her soft brown wool with the rose-beige flecks oh maybe a drop of oil or a rim of sour cream from tasting things but" she writes in her play "Trilogy."

And then Beatrice's structure on the page expresses the magical, mystical effect that Chenshe had on men, perhaps

"she

was

the

Hostess

She was not tall or willowy.

She was plump and quite stout.

Her hair was not flowing and golden.

It was bobbed and black.

She carried no magic wand.

Her efforts were so visible.

And yet

She was my fairy princess.

She was in fact… our fairy godmother.

I remember my father thought so too.

At that time

I was." Beatrice writes.

Oh, oh, oh, the woman is reeling in shock at
Chenshe's potent and magical ways.

***

With thanks to Psychiatrist Suzannah Zimmet, daughter of Beatrice Zimmet; Songstress and Counselor Marya Zimmet, daughter of Beatrice Roth; Ari Raphael Roth Zimmet, who is a Yale Graduate in the History of Art and has a Master's Degree in Social Work as well, grandson of Beatrice Roth; and Veterinarian Tech To-Be. Ava-Lily Miranda Roth Zimmet, granddaughter of Beatrice Roth. Beatrice Roth participated in the Actor's Studio with Marilyn Monroe and Marlon Brando. With thanks to Suzannah Zimmet and to Marya Zimmet for permission to use the play "The Trilogy" by Beatrice Roth, published in 1985.

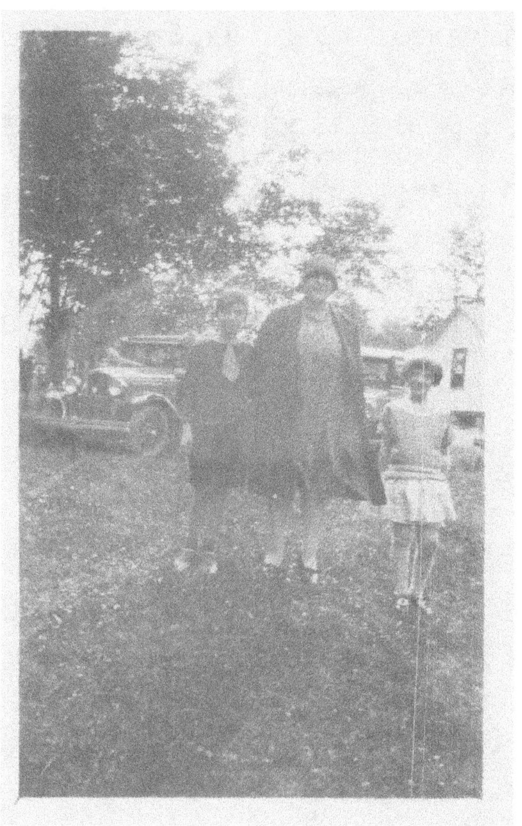

Viewed from the viewer's point of view, the picture above shows Isador's daughter, Beatrice, who was born in 1919, their Aunt Chensche, born in 1900, and Isador's daughter, Henrietta, born in 1923. The picture was taken in 1931.

After Lillie died in 1936, Beatrice, who was 17 years of age, took up Beatrice's siblings' care;

Chensche would also bring food and make clothes in 1936 when Chensche was 36 years of age.

Rosalie, the mother of Abe, Isador, and Joe, passed away in 1942, and Isador eventually married Rose Pachter in 1946 when Isador had learned of Rosalie, his mother's passing.

Ironically, Jakub, son of Bernard, who had passed in 1915, had married a sister, Serl Pachter, so when Alex Roth had taken the test, he had close relations with Pachters.

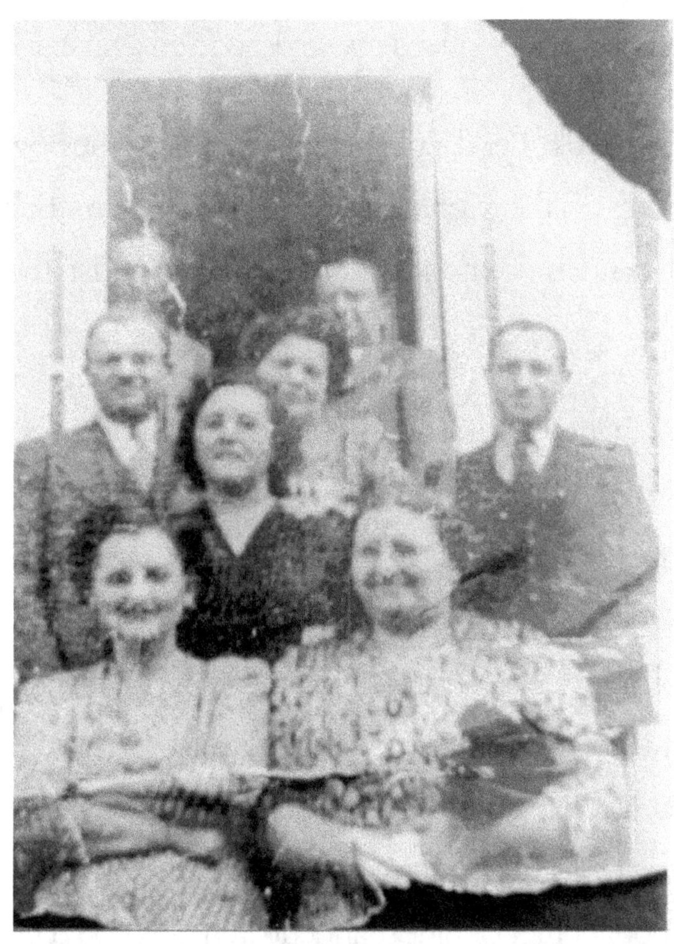

From the viewer's point of view, Isador can be seen next to his wife, Rose Pachter, in 1946, in the third row from the bottom. In 1945, a year before this picture, Chensche, who is wearing a black dress, collapsed upon learning of the news of her two sisters, one brother and wife, possibly the mother, a brother's child, a sister's two children and a husband.

Lucille, her daughter, had taken over hanging clothes on the washing line. Abe Roth, Chensche's husband, is positioned at the right-most end in the highest row.

Chensche had become like a woman of layers, a victim of historical eras, and yet she often seemed like a butterfly with her lace and silk. One era in 1945 was causing her to collapse, but there she was. In that picture, Chensche, in 1946, looks animated and ready, as if she were fascinated by life. Did she repress what had happened to her? She once let it slip "I had twelve brothers that were killed," she told a young granddaughter of nine grandchildren. She could not specifically give attention to one grandchild as she would say, "sveetheart."

Her two sons had gone to World War II; one had filed with the Red Cross to find an Alex Roth who had written a letter to Northampton. Then, in

2019, the Red Cross document was discovered by the granddaughter of Samuel Elias Roth. Samuel Elias Roth had survived Auschwitz and had written a letter in 1947. Monro had filed a document looking for Samuel Elias Roth and Samuel had not answered. Recently, a sister of Alex's has written a letter saying that her father knew about the document from the Red Cross but did not want to contact the family after he had met his future wife Maria. The sisters of Alex were also angry that his "Jewish origins" were revealed. Samuel Elias Roth, in 1947, had changed his name to Alex, the name of his aunt Berta's last child and a name of royalty.

She, being Chensche, wasn't done in life. Instead, she had a flair, a charisma, of drawing people to her as if she were an effervescent light where the butterflies were going towards the light. Her parlor on 17th Street in Allentown had groups of constant company, men and women; the woman remembers when a man, Morris or Maurice Lang, was proprietorially scolding when the woman was a child when the woman was running towards the balustrade of the stairway. Chensche's aromas of cooking included Slovakian dishes, and she had a mannequin where she sewed an outfit for each of the nine grandchildren. Monro and Harold would lay on the sofa-they were tired from their work.

Abe was ten years older, but now, with the civil document only three years older than Helen if he is born in 1897 but in the cemetery grave number he is born in 1894 which makes their age difference six years. 1984 is the accepted birth due to the cemetery stone.

Searching for Surname (phonetically like) : ROTH AND
Any Field (contains) : ZBOJ
3 matching records found.
Run on Tue, 19 Mar 2024 21:13:14 -0600

Name	Birthplace / Date of Birth / Sex	Father / Mother	Registration Town / District / County	Comments	Source / Image / Record / File
ROTH, Henrika / Chentse	Kolbaszo 110 F	ROTH, Samuel GUNCZENBERGER, Regina	Ulics Szinna Zemplén	Father age 36, grocer, b. Zboj, Mother age 29, b. Sztarina	SSA Humenne, Ulic Births Vol.02 003/1900-085 Ulics_Births_Vol02_085
ROTH, Mihaly / Melech	Kolbaszo 27-Mar-1902 M	ROTH, Samuel GUNCZENBERGER, Regina	Ulics Szinna Zemplén	Father age 37, smallholder, b. Zboj, Mother age 30, b. Sztarina	SSA Humenne, Ulic Births Vol.02 016/1902-059 Ulics_Births_Vol02_016
ROTH, Katalin	Kolbaszo 07-Jun-1904 F	ROTH, Samuel GRÜNCZBERGER, Regina	Ulics Szinna Zemplén	Father age 40, grocer, b. Zboj, Mother age 33, b. Sztarina	SSA Humenne, Ulic Births Vol.03 010/1904-097 Ulics_Births_Vol03_010

He toiled non-stop, supposedly, and they had gotten married very young. However, in 1961, Abe and Chensche had come to an understanding, according to an older granddaughter Carol. In that parlor was the grandfather's chair, where no one would sit in his chair. Then Abe and Chensche would take the children to Atlantic City and Trexler Game Preserve because this reminded them of the villages of Slovakia.

Abe passed in his early sixties. Chensche went to Florida, and she lived, danced, had an admirer whom she was now cooking for, and had a pink Thunderbird. She was the only woman who had a car, Adele said. Her brother said that Abe's furniture business was the biggest business in the state. In the 20s, cash was taken out of the business, and a Slovakian maid was living with Abe and Helen.

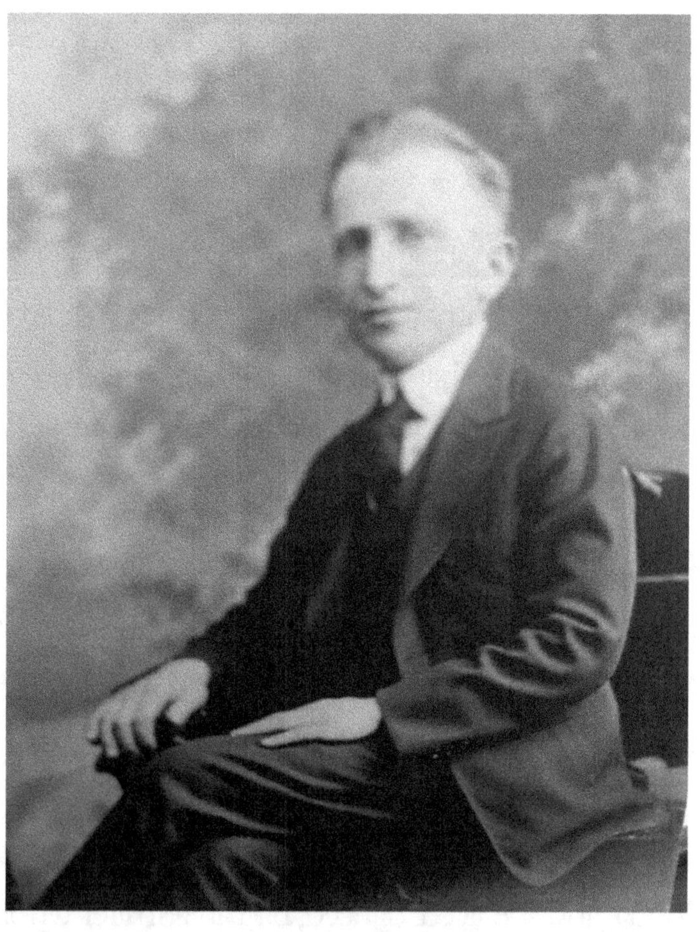

When Chensche had arrived in Northampton, Pennsylvania, in 1921, Chensche was twenty years old then, did not speak the language, lived with her uncle Isador and aunt Gunczenberger in her first year in Pennsylvania, and then she maybe had made up her mind to get married.

During the 20th century, love, friends, and staying together with relatives were all considered distant luxuries.

Abe worked day and night, supposedly, and at 23, Chensche had her first child, Monro; the name was not yet changed, in 1923. By this time, Abe was working more and more or away from the house more and more, and Chensche felt more and more isolated due to her not knowing the language. In 1924, she had her second baby, Shirley, and in 1928, she had Harold, and in 1932 she had Lucille.

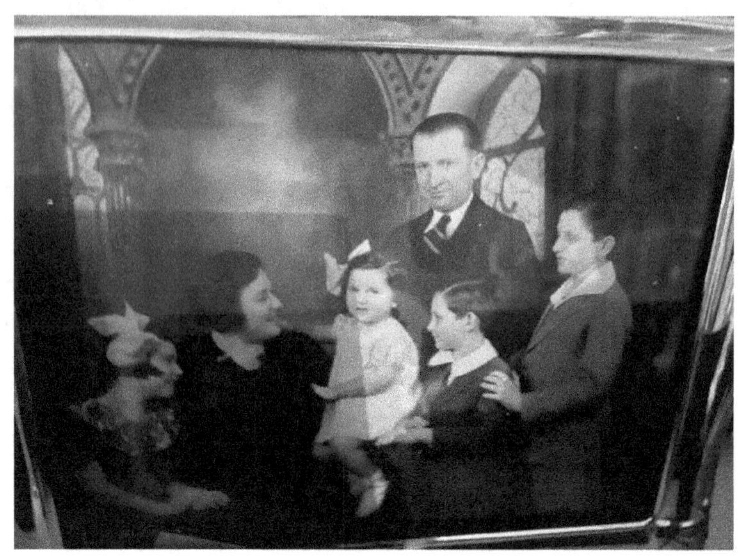

On the left is Shirley, born in 1924, and then, from the viewer's point of view, is Chensche with Lucille, born in 1932. Lucille looks to be about two years old, so the picture was taken in 1934 in Northampton, Pennsylvania, the United States. There were bows in the girls' hair, whereas in the 1936 picture of the family of Abe's in Vysna Jablonka, there were no ribbons. However, Zuzana told the story through her daughter Jana that in Vysna Jablonka, the only reason a person would leave the farm to go over to the dry goods store of the Chaimovics was to "get a ribbon or kerosene."

Zuzana remembered Bernard, the older man, sitting in that store with a white beard with the star sewn onto his shirt. Zuzana was born in 1930.

Abe, who was born in 1894, who was born in Vysna Jablonka, is in the back. He was 40 years old at that point in time when the picture was taken if the picture is in 1934. Harold, who was born in 1928, is in front of Abe and is six years old. Monro, who was born in 1923, is in front of Abe and is 11 years old. The meticulousness of the clothing, the ribbons, the wealth reflected in the background, Chensche's apparent contentment, and Abe's motivation, which is evident in his haberdashery, are the things that stand out about this picture.

Two years later, in 1936, Abe's brother, after hearing the news of impending war and threats towards groups of people, Joe Roth, born in 1897 who was 39 years old, boarded a ship and returned to Vysna Jablonka to get his sister Berta and six children. There would be three more by 1942; his brother, Jakub, had passed in 1915 of typhoid fever. Jakub had been working as a tavern keeper in Solinka and had two sons, Mor and Samuel Elias.

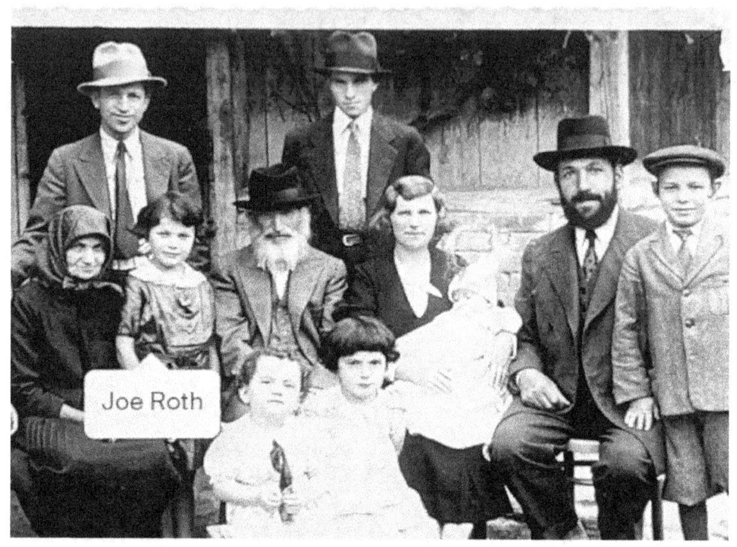

Samuel Elias, pictured in the black hat in the back row, would survive and would be discovered by his American cousins in 2019. Joe, the man in the white hat in the back row, Samuel Elias' uncle, would pose in the picture in Michalovce, Slovakia, and then would return to Allentown, Pennsylvania, after Joe had been unsuccessful in convincing his parents, his sister, his sister's six children, nine by 1942, and her husband and her brother's two sons to return to America with him.

There in that 1936 picture, the haberdashery of the outfits is also exquisite, like the picture of Abe's family in 1934. Perhaps Joe had brought the clothes, or was 1936 in Michalovce prosperous?

Looks can be accurate or deceiving; researchers often find out... 1936 opened a wellspring of events for Abe's family and also for the family of the woman Chensche, whom Abe had married.

Chensche's father had passed in 1936, and her granddaughter had made the prayer in Kolbasov's cemetery in 2022. The year after, the woman discovered that the grave was Samuel Moses Roth's.

***

The woman had stood praying while her newly discovered second cousin, who had been brought up in Teplice, Czech Republic, had said he never knew he was of a certain religion when he was a little boy. He was raised as a Christian, as his sister has written.

In 1936, there also was the loss of Lillie Weiss, who had given birth to Isador Roth's seven children. One child had written an Off-Broadway play about how Chensche had visited and cooked for Isador and his 1936 motherless seven children.

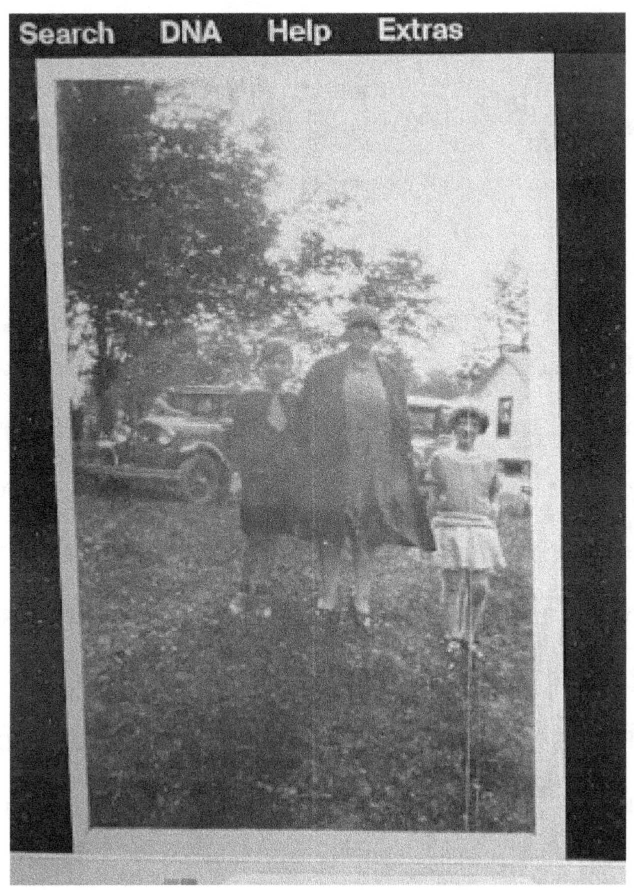

Here in the picture is Beatrice Roth with
Chensche and Henrietta Roth. The year of this
picture would be 1931 when Lillie and the outfits
were sewn by Chensche or bought. Chensche had
honed her experience by working in the tailor's shop
in the bigger city of perhaps Humenne.

The fourth event of 1936 was the abdication of the King of England for "love."

***

In 1936, Chensche was cooking and sewing and living in Northampton. Shirley said Chensche had told her that Chensche had stopped her relations after Lucille was born in 1932 because she no longer wanted children. Her husband's brother Isador had seven children with Lillie Weiss because he would not marry the woman of his life. Shirley remembers Lillie as very kind; she would often go over to the house there, Shirley said. Carol says there are no saints in the Jewish religion, but if there had been, that would be Lillie. The love of his life was Rose, the same name as his mother, Rosalie Chaimovicsova. He did not marry Rose until his mother and wife had passed due to superstition.

Chensche's father passed away and received a cemetery grave in Kolbasov. Monro said the family did not want to tell Chensche about her father's passing in 1936.

Years later, her husband Abe passed in 1961, and after that, Chensche went to Florida and danced and eventually cooked for someone as a job. Lucille is haunted by the fact that Chenshe had to work. The house of Chensche was lost by a lien. The sons were in charge of the finances. In those days, wives were often not left money. Lucille reported that Chenshe was supposed to get money from the business after 1961.

Lucille reports that Chensche and Abe used to travel by car to the Trexler Game Preserve to see the orchards because they reminded Chensche and Abe of their villages in Slovakia. Usually, they would get lost along the way to Atlantic City. Later, Abe would pass away in his sixties, and Carol, Shirley's daughter, remembers the three brothers sleeping in their chairs because they were bone tired from a day's work.

Monro Roth, in an article published in 1994, said that his parents wrote letters to their parents. Monro was in the "Air Force" in World War II and was a clerk typist for the commanding officer in Tunisia.

Later on, in 1972, when she had lost weight, Chensche told Zelda that she might need some clothes, and Zelda was surprised at what she thought was a "Sarah Bernhardt" way. Monro, in the article, says he had "dropped the woman he had been dating—Mimi—then went with a male friend," Julian Levin, to Tamiment, a Pocono mountain resort, who he describes as "a beautiful specimen arriving in a white convertible." Monro said that he was "carrying the bags for" his friend. And then Monro stated, "And there she appears, right there."

The article's writer enquired, "The same girl you dropped?"

Monro answered, "Yes, Mimi, we were married two weeks later in her mother's apartment in Washington Heights." Later, he confided that he didn't like the neighborhood or the way the area was, but then went in and met Zelda and Bea and enjoyed their warmth.

Monro then explained how, with the chains of "Levits," "the town was now empty. It happened in all the little towns," he said. He then improved his teaching with experiences of life, he said. He described his son as a "beautiful red-headed boy, born the same year our president was born... '61." He couldn't talk about this, he said, or he would cry.

He described his mother, Helen, "When it rained, she would bring the hamburgers to the school and carry them inside so that I shouldn't have to walk in the rain. You could smell the spices..." and then Monro added, "I would hide in the back row that no one should know that I belonged to her, and because of the smell of the food."

The interviewer states that she sees a black-and-white photo of a well-rounded woman smiling from the steps of a building. Is that her?" she asks. "She's lovely, don't you think so?"

Monro responded, "Now I do."

Monro explained then that he had lived in Northampton from 1923 until 1943. The Nieman sisters went to get teenage Abe in what Monro called Hungary and explained that it was Hungary until 1917.

Monro explained that Helen came in 1921 and that she was a store clerk for the Gunczenbergers in Northampton. They had a five-and-dime store.

Monro said that Abe was "thirty and she was twenty," although the woman believed they were six years apart due to the cemetery record and her civil record they are 29 and 23, according to the Slovak civil record, which revealed Helen's date of birth as 1900 but with Abe being born in 1894, then there was a six- year difference.. He stated that they "immediately fell in love after they discovered they weren't related. This was 1922," he added.

Monro described Northampton, which "was very small. There was no synagogue." Lucille said there was a Schul on Washington Avenue.

Lance Flax, whose father was good friends with Harold, described Northampton like this: *"In Northampton, there was the Newport area." There was "the other side of the railroad tracks." He explains that there was an area between the railroad and the river.*

But the main street was Newport Avenue, he explained.

Lance Flax's father was Leon Flaxgold. Later on, he had a billboard business, which had "nothing to do with Northampton."

His father had a store.

His great-grandfather on his mother's side had a store at 14ᵗʰ Street at Newport

Avenue.

Lance Flax goes on to say, "They had come to the country as Koslosky from Courtland, Lithuania in 1872, which was a part of Russia then."

There was a relative in Reading, a family from Reading Leon Miller, who lent money.

As they got settled, they decided to go to the coal area, Lance Flax explains.

"They moved to Lansford and had a store for coal miners." Lance Flax explained.

Lansford was east of Manchunk, Jim Thorpe, and Tamaqua.

The family left there in the 1900's and moved to 14th and Newport Avenue in Northampton, Pennsylvania. Morris Frank served with Roosevelt in the Spanish-American war in 1898.

Lance Flax's father's uncle was a bootlegger and was involved in gambling, what Lance Flax refers to as "the black sheep."

In 1953, the store was sold, and his grandfather retired and bought a house on Glenwood Street in Allentown.

Leon Flaxgold was good friends with Harold the son of Abe. Leon, who was 6 foot 3, was a good athlete, and a scout came and asked whether he would like to play baseball. He decided instead to go to Penn State. Harold wanted to visit Leon Goldflax across the tracks, but after being beat up by the guys there, Harold had a new strategy of yelling across the tracks, "Come meet me across the railroad tracks."

Lance Flax then told the end of this story which was this - after World War II, "Everyone had served." - Both sides of guys on both sides of the railroad tracks no longer fought each other.

Due to the fact that all who had served in World War II, with guys from both sides

***of the railroad tracks- they no longer beat
each other up or harassed each other.***

Harold's older brother continued within his
article published in 1994 about his parents, "They
went to Scranton to get married." He adds they did
this because she had the two brothers there, Max and
Harry.

Nine months later, Monro said, he "was born in
the apartment over the store."

Monro explained that he learned how to read by
spreading out the "funnies from the newspaper" on
the front porch, and the funnies were "very colorful."

He reported that he was "hyper" and could not
sit still. In first grade in 1930, he "sat behind a girl
named Lorraine," and then he said, "On my desk
was a pen with an inkwell in the corner."

Monro said, "In those days, everyone wanted to
look like Shirley Temple. When the teacher said
something amusing, Lorraine's curls would move

back and forth before me. 'Wouldn't it be wonderful to dip them in ink?'"'

His teacher, who was six feet tall, Miss Gochenbach, was mad with the ink dipping and the drawing on the walls. In twelve years, he was the only Jewish child. He added, "If anything came up involving someone who was Jewish, everyone would turn and look at me."

Monro would then think, "'If only I could be Pennsylvania Deutsch. It would solve everything.'"

He explains that there were 13 Jewish families in the town of Northampton of 10,000 people. A few were ragmen or peddlers. He added, "This is how I spent my youth: looking at the trains with a hundred cars." After Monro had seen the acclaimed movie "Nebraska," where a man just pulled up a chair and watched the cars go by, Monro recalled how some people in Northampton would pull up a chair and watch the train go by.

A furniture owner, Mr. Glazier, was determined to get a minyan. That is the number of ten people who were supposed to make the praying holy. Women were not permitted. Some people left for the minyan from their stores, Monro explained.

"The families were mostly from Eastern Europe-Hungary, Czechoslovakia. The people from Hungary spoke no Yiddish and came from small villages with little education," he added.

When Monro was asked about Torah study, he said, "A rabbi came from a village and had a cheder - a school. He had ten children, his name was Roth, and he had a contract for 10 dollars." This Roth was Berta Roth and brother Leon Roth's father, who was related to Chensche as third cousins. He added, "It was understood that his house be available to any itinerant collectors for the Yeshivas in Palestine. Without knowing English, without a driver's license, they came." Monro added, "They would not get out of the store until they got 18 dollars." The Chai in

Hebrew meant life or good luck or eighteen.

Leon Roth later explained what growing up in a village near Kolbasov was like. Later, in the United States, he became a building contractor, but in Slovakia, as a boy, he was very scrawny and would walk to a guest house and eat chicken on Saturday, which was considered very special.

Morris Gunczenberger was helped by Leon's father to immigrate, as dictated by Morris Gunczenberger-"*Rabbi Morris Roth was a friend from Europe." He sponsored Maurice Gunszenberger." Morris continued," "He tried to get out from 1935 until 1938. Eventually, he came this way: he promised an uncle's son that he was trustworthy. He traveled by train to Nuremberg, then Paris, then Cherbourg. He recalls that many Nazis got on the train in Nuremberg. He was met at the boat by Aunt Jenny Gladstone who was Rifka Gunczenbergers's sister. He says they looked poor and shabby, and he remembers that he felt depressed and wanted to go back to Slovakia."* He came late and was on the train with the Nazis. According to Monro, he was handsome and would say, "Spielen den ball."

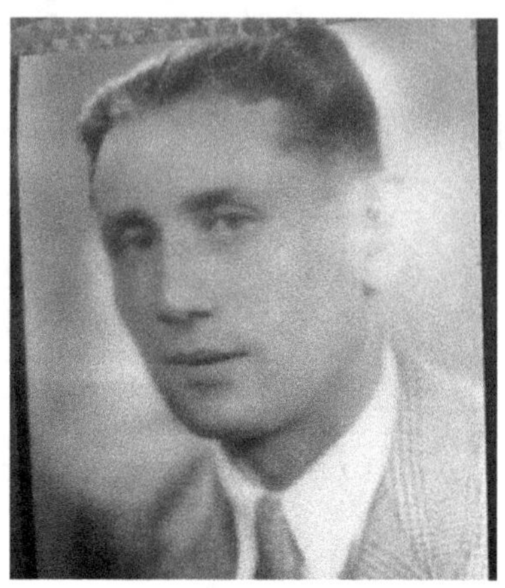

Outside in Northampton. Morris Gunczenberger came late when the war had begun, and somehow, he got through a train ride with Nazis on it. He would work for Mr. Weinstein, whose son would later own Dorney Park. As dictated by Morris Gunczenberger: *"Helen Roth came from Northampton, Pennsylvania, to New York and brought Morris back to Northampton. He got a job at a shirt factory which Isador Weinstein owned. Morris was* given a pile of shirts to sew on button holes. He *sewed the button holes on the wrong side and did a large pile of shirts this way. Mr.* Weinstein *threw the pile back at him, and Morris quit,"* said Lucille. *"He lived with*

Helen Roth and insisted on paying 5 to 8 dollars to Helen.
When he returned to New York, Helen gave him back the
money."

Morris remembered in his dictation "telling Lucille that
Helen was 'very beautiful.'" There was a general postmaster, a
non-Jew, in the town, and he was very much in love with
Mother," Lucille said. "Jennie worked in the Rosner Hotel."
Harris Weinstein, with the anecdote at his funeral, a
person told how he had respected all his workers.
When asked how he knew Prince Andrew, he had
said, "Not from Hebrew school," but in his father's
factory, Morris had sewed the buttons wrong, and
the boss threw the shirts at him, and he threw them
back and then Morris went to New York to go into
jewelry with his in-laws.

Monro reported, too that he "might have to say"
to the religious solicitors, "My father's not here. You'll
have to come back. They would not get out.
Sometimes, they spoke only Yiddish. They would
say 'heaven waits you' if you give money to take care

of poor people."

The interviewer then asked Monro Roth if they were "legitimate," and Monro responded, "There were no details," and then he added;

"You have to have faith."

In the bed, as a child, Monro's mother, Chensche in Kolbasov, probably shared that with her siblings from babyhood on, her bare feet walked anywhere she wanted to go, and that was rarely to school. The expelled "Traveling People" had become her friends and some boyfriends. Morris dictated to Lucille that he, as a child, was "living in a kibbutz with bunk beds in a big barn" during the 1930's. In Sztarina, "the children made bricks. Europe was mobilizing. He worked from Friday until Wednesday. Young people were also mobilizing." Morris, who was the nephew of Rifka Gunczenberger, added, "As early as 1935, Zionists knew trouble was coming. Morris spoke about a joint committee trying to get children out of Europe in 1938." He added that Czechoslovakia never thought that Chamberlain would give away Czechoslovakia. He stopped to see Helen's brother and sisters in September of 1938.

Morris' dictation continues: he "wrote to Rabbi Roth, Leon Roth's father. Herb Hyman's grandfather who was the schoicet, who killed chickens in a kosher religious ritual in Northampton, Pennsylvania., to sponsor Morris." Herb Hyman was the grandson of Yecheil Chaimovics. Ironically, Herb Hyman's son Nat Hyman has just purchased the Beer Brewery in Northampton, Pennsylvania, as of October 2024.

Chensche's mother, Rifka, was hardscrabble from giving birth to babies in the small house with two rooms. The relief was when Chensche could work at the tavern in Sztarina at 15 years old in 1915, but she would stride there with bare feet. At 20, she got the idea that she could go to America, where it

was rumored that the streets were "paved with gold,"
according to Anna Chaimovicsova Nieman, as told
by her daughters Bertha and Edith. "She went to
Prague alone by train," according to Lucille; "she was
sad to leave her mother and father," Lucille said.

She chose to wed 29-year-old Abe when she
was 23 years old—her age is according to the
Slovakian civil record, although Monro states that
Abe was 30 and Chensche 20, and they moved to a
home in Northampton with a Slovakian maid.

Adele's husband smoked a cigar, drank a glass of
alcohol in a sunken den in Allentown, Pennsylvania,
and gave an opinion of them in 2020. He said that
"the children raised themselves."

There were four children before she decided she
didn't want any more. After the war, in 1946, her
husband moved the family to 17th Street, where
many people passed by on their way to the temple
and entered Chensche's parlor. Adele's husband said

Chensche's husband was constantly grooming with posh clothes, barber hairdos, and manicures. Adele's brother said Chensche's husband and Chensche's younger son were wild. "Wild" meant philandering and gambling. She was sewing and cooking, when in Northampton, she aimed to take the trolley daily to Allentown, Pennsylvania, Shirley said. While living in Northampton, she wanted to go where Hess' Department store was, Shirley said. One day, Chensche and Abe walked into the burlesque and saw their son Harold cutting school, Adele said. In fact, Chensche's parlor had become a thing of excitement; men would gather. Once, a second cousin to Abe had become a doctor, Herb Chaimovics, Yecheil's grandson, and he would enter and go right to the refrigerator.

The secret of Chenshe was revealed: Her first son's daughter was tested in Ancestry. The second daughter's daughter was tested in Ancestry and she turned out to be not from the husband. The daughter of the second daughter called and revealed:

In childhood, the father of the second child approached the second child and said, "I am your father." *The second child had a problem throughout life with impulse control and getting along with people and perhaps if the siblings had heard from this second daughter that she was not from the husband - perhaps the siblings did not believe this second child.*

Ironically, the second child's father had a son who became an acclaimed poet from two acclaimed universities, and the first son of Chensche always had admired this poet. In fact, the first son, called the university and spoke with the poet and got the second daughter an admittance into that university.

The third child had three children, and none were willing to take the Ancestry test. The wife of the third child had taken the children down to Florida and the children were a bit remote with the needs of other requests.

The fourth child was from the husband.

The explanation from the second child's daughter was this: Chensche did not know the language and felt isolated in Northampton. Meanwhile, her husband, according to the husband's brother's son, Barry, was gambling and "wild," which meant that he had other women. The couple apparently was ill-suited for each other. In addition to this, Chenshe's husband's brother, who had lost his wife in 1936, had fallen in love with Chenshe. However, this was later on, but in 1924, Chenshe was isolated and away from her Slovakian family. The daughter of the second child of Chenshe also said that Chenshe was isolated due to Chenshe not knowing English.

The first child, a son, said that Chenshe and her

husband were constantly bickering. They were six years apart, if one uses the cemetery stone as a source, although it was interpreted that the two had a large age gap between each other.

Later on, with the fourth child who was definitively from the husband, and according to the daughter of the second child, the couple Chenshe and her husband had come to an understanding.

The amazing thing is that Chenshe had performed as if she were going to get an Academy Award, and no one knew about this other child's identity, and yet, at one high holiday, the second daughter of Chenshe and Chenshe herself were squabbling in the kitchen while the little daughters and wife of the first son of Chenshe were witness to that. Chenshe was quietly weeping in the kitchen with her second child in about 1964.

Chenshe had been through many eras of history

and many settings of different countries, and now she was performing. . . throughout her life as she dissembled to her children and husband. . .

One day, the family received a telephone, and Monro screamed into the telephone, according to his own story. He was told he did not have to scream in order to speak on the telephone. Helen would play later cards on the porch with female companions. Later on, she would drive a pink Thunderbird in Florida and walk the boardwalks as she had in Atlantic City in her lace and silk.

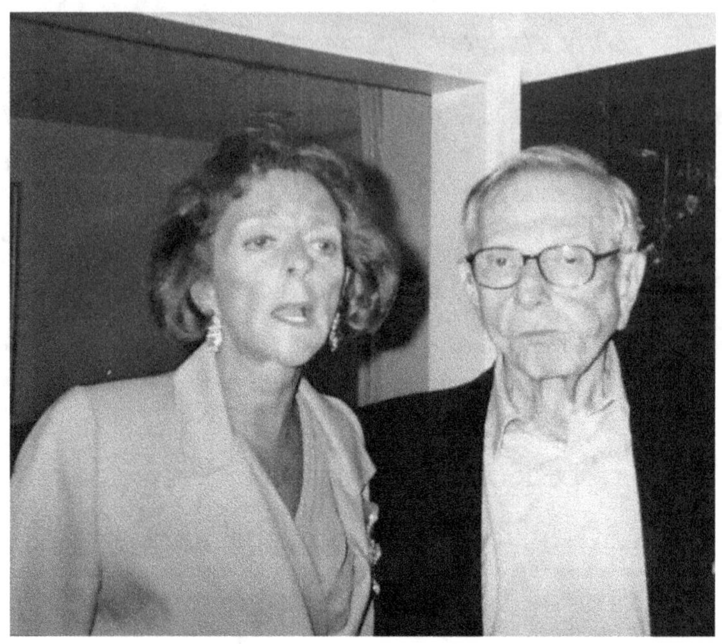

Abe and Helen's relatives would stop by, go to the refrigerator, and eat something. He became a doctor. His wife is a colorful entrepreneur of jewelry and purses. That is M. Lauder and Herb Chaimovics the grandson of Yecheil Chaimovics. There also was a Mr. and Mrs. Schneider, a Morris Lang and Yolan Feldman Lang.

In Allentown, the meeting place was the diner patterned after a railcar run by Greek workers. The same one hundred dollars went around the town, and some philanthropists like Max Hess, owner of Hess's Store, eventually helped support community centers and religious places of worship. Since Berta Roth Chaimovicsova married to Elmore, lived to be 98 years old, Berta was called by Monro, and Berta said bitterly that Chenshe danced at the Jewish Community Center, and some felt snubbed by her.

In Allentown, the woman did feel the hierarchy of the manufacturers' children, yet she had three companions, one was the niece of a factory owner, Gerson Lazar, who had begun with one sewing machine, his wife told Monro Roth. Esther, his wife, waited on Monro and made the food that his mother Chenshe had made as Monro helped to write a speech for Gerson, and Esther cried. Once, in the synagogue, Mimi and the woman watched as people went by with a carpet bent, and suddenly Gerson straightened out the carpet, and Mimi said, "And now you know why he is a successful business man. The other companion was Jane who walked to covered bridges with the woman. Jane went on to write plays and married a cousin of John Singer Sargeant. The other good friend was a great-niece of Joey Bishop who was head of the "Rat Pack." Joey Bishop, in a comedy routine, saw Marilyn Monroe enter, and he said, "I told you to wait in the truck."

Still there was materialism and a hierarchy amidst the flourishing of the factories and yet the townspeople sorely miss that prosperity.

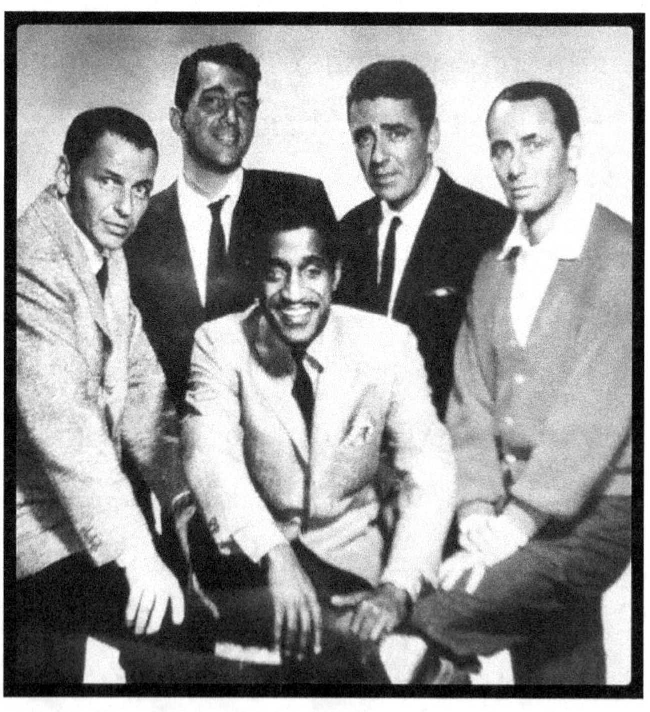

This Photo by Unknown Author is licensed under CC BY-SA-NC

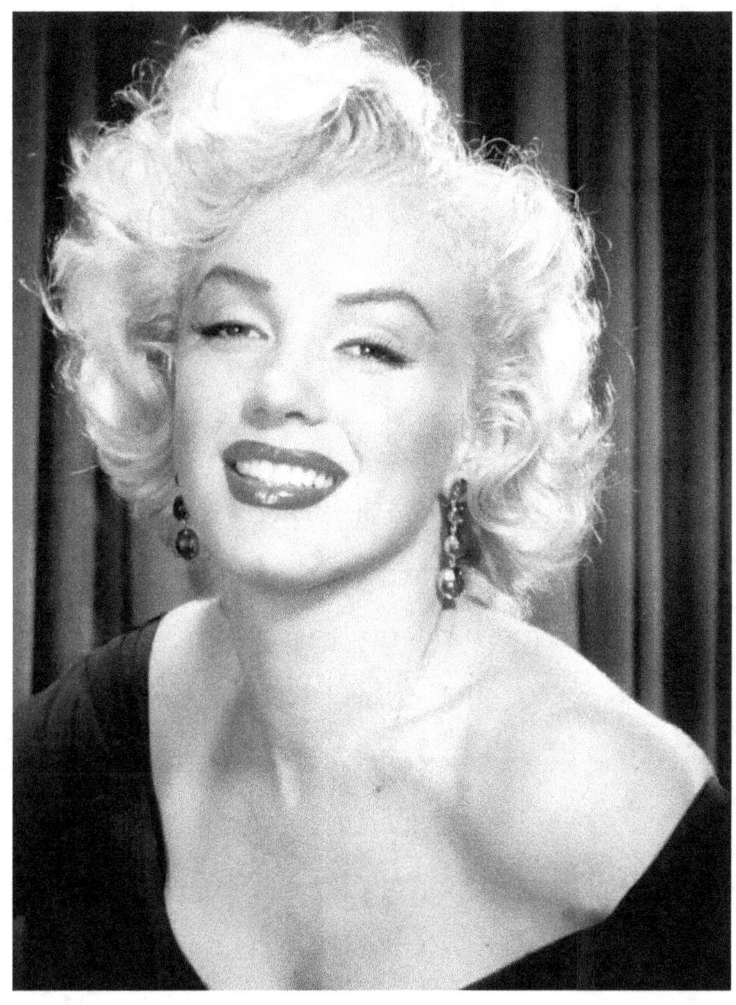

Mimi reported that the same hundred dollars

was circulated around the town and opened factories

in the 1950s after World War II had decimated

businesses in Europe. According to a business columnist, life was prosperous due to the factories in Germany and Japan being down. Children walked the streets safely and explored the woods but stayed on the street paths. The children also walked to the covered bridges the German-descent farmers had built.

The anchors of Allentown were the diner, churches, mostly Lutheran, with all services in German in the 1800s due to the German-descent farmers, later Catholics, and the synagogues, which often had the businessmen of Northampton, which were Orthodox, Conservative, and Reform. Art schools, dance schools, and community centers were also anchors. There were holocaust survivors who were Hebrew school teachers in Allentown. There also were many interfaith groups and life was peaceful. Yiddish speakers were able to understand Pennsylvania Deutsch says many residents of Allentown, Pennsylvania.

The miraculous beauty of finding relatives in the Czech Republic is Alex Roth, Jr. and his six siblings, families from Samuel Elias Roth son of Jakub son of Bernard.

Bernard Roth	Roza Chajmovic Roth
Jakub/Abe/Isador/Joe/Berta	

Samuel Elias Roth had survived.

Another joy was from finding the two out-of-wedlock children, Mary, grandmother of Francis, and Michael, father of Zuzana, from a first cousin of the woman's great-grandmother.

But then it happened again. Some more shocks of the study of history.

Amidst the stumbling of mankind, womenkind, the straying, the money taken out of business, the gambling, the losses, the alliances-another liaison was discovered of Izrael Chaimovics. And then another alliance that made these four children. From three alliances, Jan Augusta suggested that Dave Lawrence Lucas from Emporium, Pennsylvania, was a great-grandson of Izrael Chaimovic.

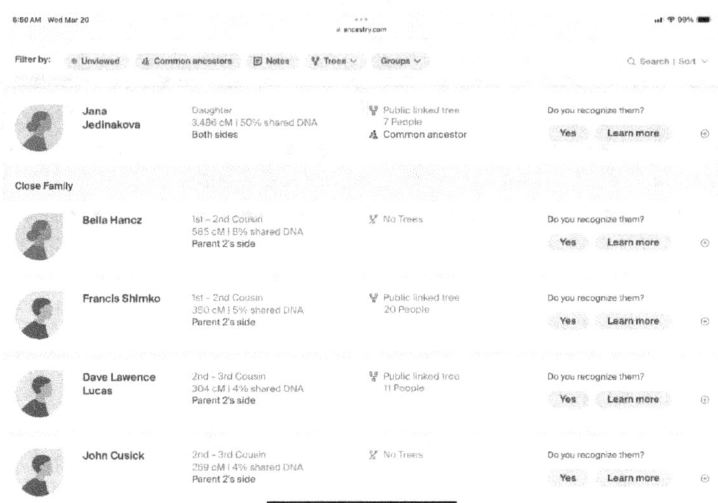

The Centimorgans fit in perfectly, the ethnic composition with a difference in Scottish for his mother. This was discovered six years later on the 4 of December 2023. DIAGRAM OF IZRAEL'S CHILDREN FROM ALLIANCES

Izrael-Tatiana	Izrael Chaimovic-Sofia	Izrael -Maria
Maria Gula	Michael/Mary	John

Father	Zuzana/Helen	Ray
John Cusick	Jana/Francis	Dave L.L.

DIAGRAM OF IZRAEL'S ALLIANCES' FOLLOWING GENERATIONS-JOHN CUSICK, JANA, FRANCIS, AND DAVE LAWRENCE LUCAS HAVE ALL ANCESTRY TESTED.

Now, Izrael Chaimovics had to be thought about seriously.

What had happened?

Izrael was born in 1858. He was a businessman and prosperous – his children were:

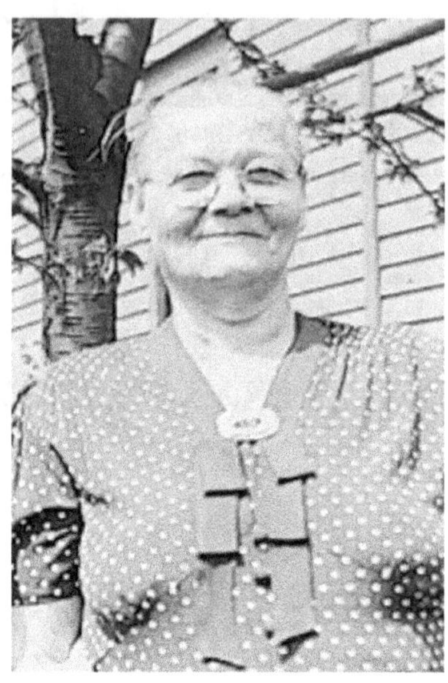

1) Mary Gula was born in 1878 from Tatiana and Izrael Chaimovics. According to the Centimorgans of a great-grandson, John Cusick, there is a high percentage that John was a half-first cousin once removed to Zuzana, with a different grandmother than Zuzana's. John Cusick was a General in the Vietnam War. John Williams, a nephew of John Cusick, reported that Mary Gula was illegitimate.

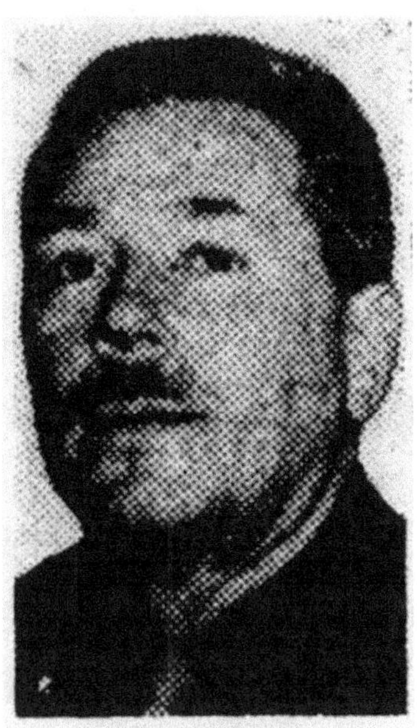

2) John Lawrence was born to Maria Babics in 1890—the great-grandson Dave Lawrence Lucas, whose great-grandfather is Izrael. Dave had written that there had been a lot of secrets in his family. Meanwhile, his grandfather had been in a Korean prison camp and was the son of Izrael Chaimovics.

Here, Izrael had a different alliance with Maria Babics, and the Centimorgans had a high percentage that Dave Lawrence Lucas, too, was a half-first cousin once removed to Zuzana.

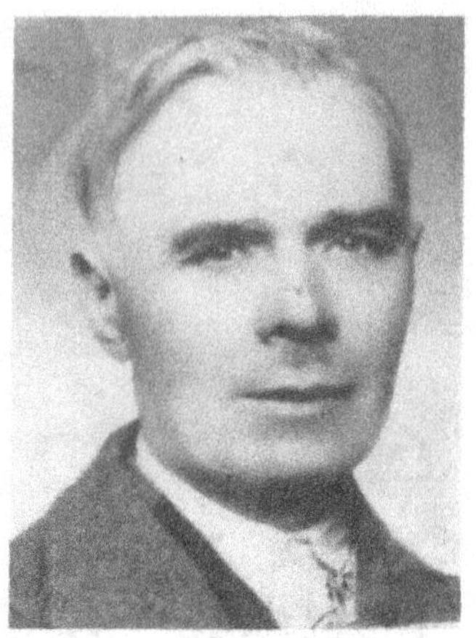

3) Michael Kunco was born in 1896 from Sofia Gula.

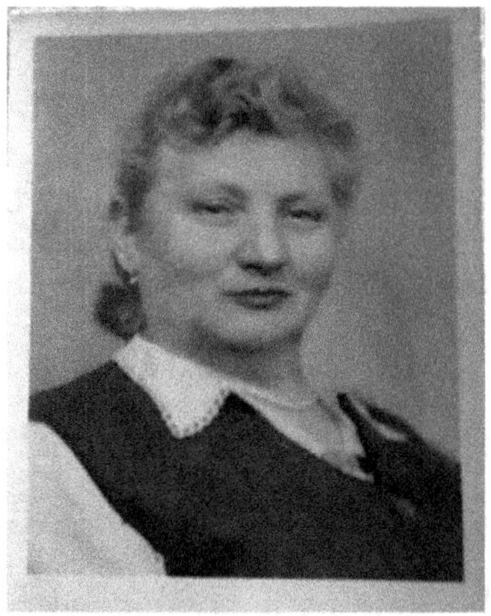

4) Leah was born in 1897 from wife Rachel. Leah emigrated to Canada.

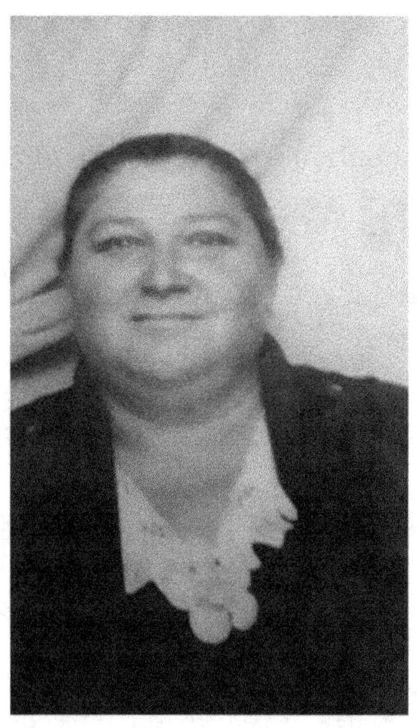

5) Mary Kunso was born in 1900 from Sofia Gula.

6) Jakub Chaimovics was born in 1904. Izrael would reside with this son in the 1930 Census in Humenne. Jakub was listed with his parents-in-law. There was a Rosalie Chaimovics, born in 1913 from Vysna Jablonka. The woman is assuming that this might have been an alliance for Izrael. Izrael's wife Rachel had passed in 1925 with an identified grave. Jakub and his family apparently did not survive. There were two daughters and a wife. Izrael passed before the

Shoah.

Jakob was the shock for the woman. She was reminded of her time as a teacher in the inner-city schools. Dear reader, in one school in North Philadelphia, a woman in "Benjamin Franklin High School" was asked to get food from a truck and brought food to two boys who asked. They did not want to go to the cafeteria for that food. One guard approached the woman and told her she did not have to do that. That guard, a success in that world, had eleven children with several "baby mamas" - that is the non-mainstream dialect term. After the woman had the student with the flicker and a foot-high flame and the woman threw the Tennessee Williams' book on the flame in that same school, she called the guard after that whenever there was a flicker of a lighter. The woman, with Izrael Chaimovics and his children, also recalled another gentleman who was a cook with eleven children who cooked for "Midtown" restaurant in Philadelphia until 2020. When asked how many "baby mamas" he had,

Elton, the cook, had to pause to think. He had five. He had picked cotton in Mississippi, so he said that he could work all day standing due to the picking of cotton.

Elton had been offered a full football scholarship at Mississippi College. He was fiercely against abortion and supported Republican Donald Trump.

The guard and Elton were both African American, charming, hard working with many children.

The woman sat in that restaurant, read three newspapers, and then gave them to Elton. He would inquire why she would underline. When she was exasperated at her job, he tried to comfort her.

Thinking of Elton, the cook, and the other, the guard of "Benjamin Franklin High School" was a reminder of how the situation of Izrael Chaimovics and these men were similar.

In psychobiology, when the tree is about to die, seeds are shed in a very abundant amount. Within this theory, psychologists suggest a theory for people who feel a danger of possible morbidity. Izrael had three different women other than his wife, so far discovered, with four children from three alliances and two children from his wife, one of whom, Jakub, did not survive, another Hersdiek, a birth mortality. The three alliances were within three blocks of Vysna Jablonka. Izrael Chaimovics was a prosperous businessman with land and horses and was taking eggs and sheep to the bigger town of Humenne. As Izrael Chaimovics' brother Yecheil's great-grandson Marshal Hyman in 2024 at a party for Alex Roth, Jr. in Allentown, Pennsylvania said, when Marshal was told about Izrael's three alliances-Marshal a Washington attorney and accountant-not missing a beat-asked, ''What was Izrael's opening line?''

But the woman began to recall when she was upset about Michael. She had bought him a Remy jacket made in America, a ''proud'' literary device of figurative language - "pathetic fallacy-ascribing an emotion to an inanimate thing"- for her, for 200 hundred dollars at a place called Torres, a store where large athletes went when he already was going to the bars daily with Diana, the rental agent, and as the woman traveled back from Atlantic City on her monthly occasion, she began to tell her story of Michael and the rental agent Diana to a woman on the bus. The woman who was African American on the bus said that women who were African American usually did not have time to be lovesick and that Michael was probably sitting at the posh bar "Rouge" next to the apartment building where he worked where the woman lived. Sure enough, he was sitting in the Remy jacket with the rental agent.

The remnants of the distress of the history of the United States still have effects. The students used to ask, "Are you black or white?" Another teacher said as the boundaries became blurred, the identities became different. She often being "the other" - the minority was dubbed "white lady," "snowflake," or "snow white," she recalled, as she wondered about Izrael Chaimovics and Abe and Chensche Roth. The other alliance was Nathan Weiss, who had a son, Ted Weiss, a poet and scholar. He was the father of the second child. Ted's wife was a musician, and they often had home shows in their row home in Allentown. Sadly, Nathan fell off a horse in 1945. *He was Chenshe's baby daddy for baby number two and maybe baby number three and their half- brother was a famous scholar, Ted Weiss. Maybe she went to the sanitarium for that loss as well.*

With victories of working this all out though - like a crossword puzzle - was this: the woman could write by email and question Jana, her newly discovered fourth cousin whose uncle Jan Kunco lived in the village of Vysna Jablonka in Slovakia. She could ask Jana to ask Zuzana, "Did the Jewish people know where they were going in the village?" and "How did the people get water?"

In "The History of Hapsburg Jews 1670-1918,"

written by William O. McCagg Jr., published by Library of Congress in 1989 ISBN 0253-33189-7, on p. 202, Dr. McCagg writes, "In northern and especially in northeastern Hungary, however, in what later became the Sub-Carpathian Ukraine, one encountered communities which by western Jewish standards had hardly changed since 'medieval times.'"

The blessing is that Jana wrote back and queried her mother Zuzana and sometimes her uncle Jan Kunco, who lived in Vysna Jablonka where Bernard Roth had lived, and nothing has changed; there is a cheese churner, a farm of chickens, and Slovakian decorations on the walls.

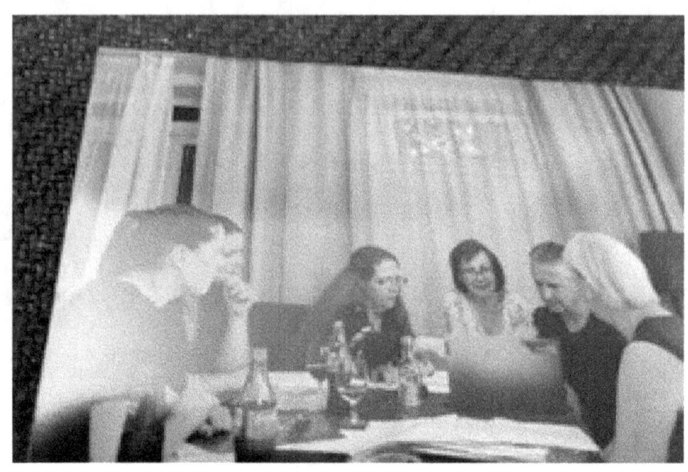

The picture contains from the left, viewer's point of view-Kata, Jr., Sona daughter of Alex, Jr., Melinda, Jana, Vlad, and Ursula in a Humenne hotel which costs 58 dollars per night., Ursula is the wife of Alex Jr.

Jana answered the woman's questions that the water had to be brought in by wooden vats in the winter, and in summer, the residents of Vysna Jablonka swam in the streams.

As for the Jewish people, according to Zuzana, Jana reports that people thought that the Jewish people were going to labor camps for work.

The miracle of seeing Alex Roth, the woman's second cousin, after her father had looked for his father in 1947 after Samuel Elias had written a letter and then went to Teplice, Czech Republic, to live with an army buddy, a miracle is his son Alex Roth, Jr.'s eyes and his character traits which remind the woman of her father Monro Roth and similarities also to Harold Roth, the brother.

Meanwhile, Jimmy Shapiro first cousin to Mimi Roth, Zelda's brother Morris' son, had two children who were unknown to the relatives until 2019. A letter had been written by his father's sister, Rose's son's wife, about Jimmy, son of Morris Shapiro, son of Max Shapiro. **"To us, his life was so glamorous," and "we spent a truly memorable afternoon with him. To us, he was a romantic figure."**

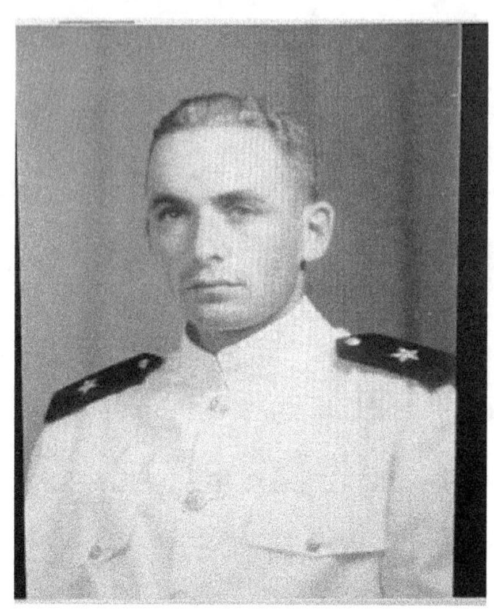

"Living all over the world, flying planes including for William Holden, brokering airplane sales. But Jimmy confessed to us, to our amazement that he felt he had been a disappointment to the family. He felt that Richard," Rose Stern's son - Rose was the sister of Zelda, "had led the life he was supposed to have led - the conventional one: college, law school, marriage to the nice Jewish girl. Practicing law, living in the New York City suburbs, raising Jewish children. . . we were astounded that he had felt this way, when, to us,

his life was so glamorous. Anyway, not long after that, maybe a few months, he passed."

Monro, son of Abe, worked with his brother Harold at "Roth Brothers" in Northampton. Outside of Allentown, and then in 1970, he worked as an English professor until he was 91 and passed at 92. Harold worked at his furniture store until he was 87.

Monro had a card that said, "Have speech, will travel." Mimi said Helen had said that Mimi had "bewitched" Monro when he had finally decided to marry at thirty. Mimi had told her daughter "to marry a best friend." Instead, perhaps the bad boy and not the nice guy, she had been involved with. The daughter did not yet take that advice. Bea and Sylvia followed Isaac Bachevis Singer, who wrote about the supernatural spirituality of Eastern Europe mostly. They followed him on the bus in New York City after he gave a talk. Edith and Bertha Nieman brought over Abe. Sandy, Harold's woman friend, when previously asked about her son and his girlfriend, bent her elbow and said, "They're both druggies, they deserve each other."

Alex had built his shoe holder where shoes were taken off before coming into houses and apartments, and he had built his children's kitchens as he did others. Monro was always reading and preparing. Samuel Elias, who survived, had been in the Czech Republic and was working on carpentry, as did Alex Roth, Jr. in the Czech Republic. He reminded the woman of her father.

Baruch Hashem means blessed is the name. Each time a salesman would come to "The Roth Brothers" furniture store in Northampton if he were religious, the man would say, "Baruch Hashem, will you sell these light fixtures?"

But the woman realized that reality, romance, and narrative were not always in sync. The grandparents from the different villages; well, one came later, another came earlier, and Abe bought insurance policies for parents in the village and Joe was heartbroken over that, Barry, Joe's son, said. Joe said that Abe and Harold did gambling and there were wild ways, other liaisons. . . money being taken out of the business. Then there was the great-grandmother's first cousin, Izrael Chaimovics, who had three different alliances with different women and four children outside of marriage and four great-grandchildren discovered through Ancestry and wondering whether these liaisons were through the barter system of romance or need.

One of Izrael's children, Michael Kunco, was told by relatives, as reported by Jana, "*She remembers that she used to go to the store. She remembers that those who sold there took turns- about three people. I think that Sophia and his lover*" (sic) "*met in the store.*" Jana's cousin continued, "*Last Sunday my cousin Michael was with us and we told about you and family Roth from Czech Republic about your visit. He is 75 years old, he grew up in Vysna Jablonka. He said that our grandfather*" (Michael Kunco son of Israel Chaimovic "*was different from the other men in the village, because he was more domineering, more cultured like the others," "men in the village, he did not act as a peasant, he also dressed more lordly and he was prudent." Both, the peasants and the leaders, were respected, yet what was interesting was the attitude of the people.*

Then, finally, the woman who was blessed to find a second cousin was told that other second cousins did not want to meet due to their discovery of their relative's "origins" and, of course, ironically, their own "origins." Everything was not always what it seemed, yet the resilience of Alex, Sona, Vladimir, and Ursula, who insisted upon meeting the American relatives, gave great hope to humans.

Hermina Gunczenberger's granddaughter Linda Fenster wrote a sympathy note to Mimi regarding Monro in 2015: "As children, Helene and I" the granddaughter of Hermina and Henrik Gunczenberger, "couldn't wait to see cousin Helen and Abe and their family, to explore their newly decorated rooms. . ."

The granddaughter of Henrik who was brother to Rifka Gunczenberger, said, "Monro was my ideal. He was young, freckle-faced with an infectious smile, and could play the guitar and sing! What perfection! . . . you loved in return! You were the Disneyland of relatives."

Monro described in an article the devotion of his mother, the fetching of Abe by Edith and Bertha Nieman when Abe was 16, although the numbers for his date of birth might indicate 13. Monro also described how he grew up looking at the train tracks. He also explained wanting to be a Pennsylvania Deutsch in Northampton.

Also, Vlada said the statement "I still love my Jewish wife" so eloquently after other siblings of Alex did not want to meet the American cousins because of the discovery of the Americans' "origins" - one could place the name of the "Other," whoever was left out of the other people's groups. This statement was made by one of the relatives. However, the woman considers thanks to God and to the freedom of the United States, perhaps, and was grateful to consider these "origins" as a religion for her.

To Vladimir saying, "I still love my ___________wife," where the underline symbolizes "The Other," "The Excluded Group" was the clarion call, the plea for humans to have humanity towards all groups. And the woman would make peace with the second cousins, Alex's siblings, by writing a very conciliatory letter. And thus, humanity will have its clarion call. . .

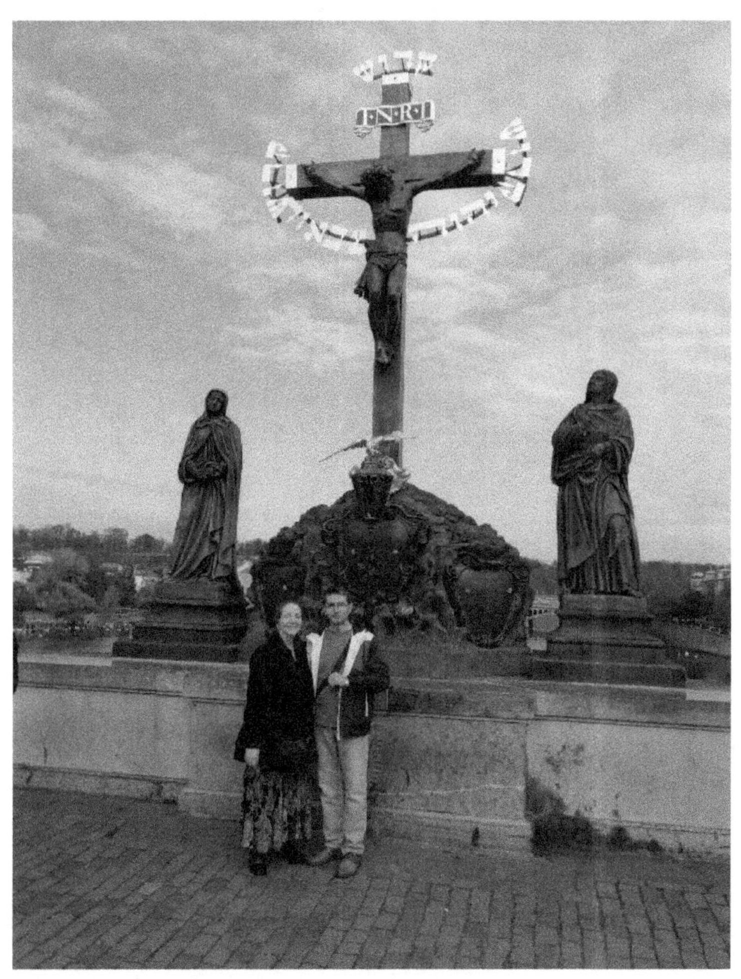

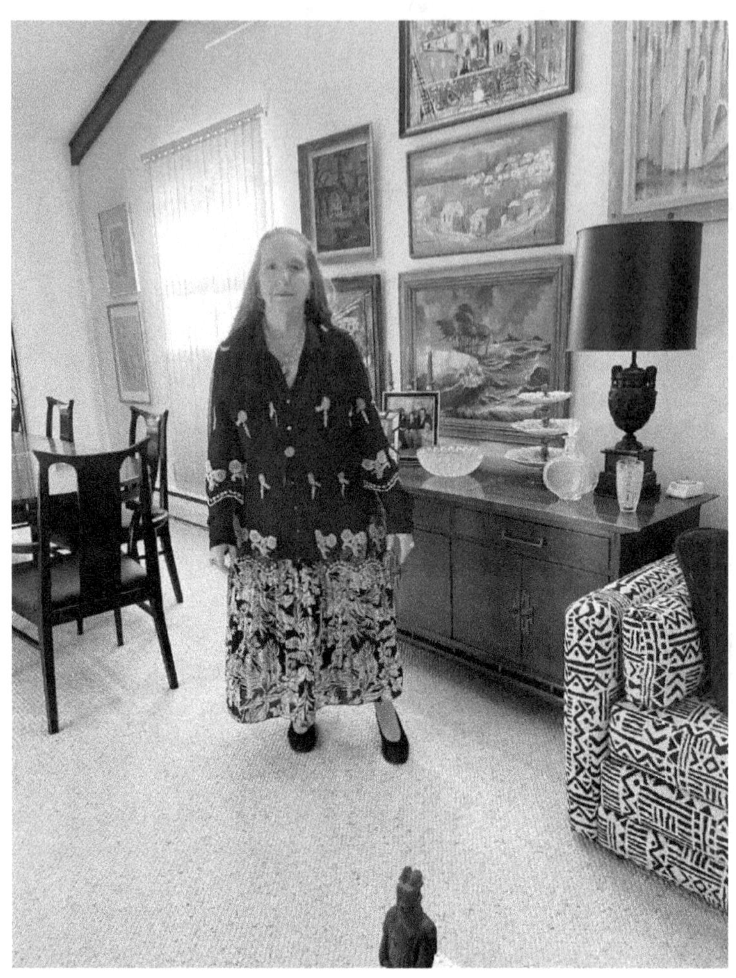